HOW TO LIVE TO BE 100

HOW TO LIVE TO BE 100

Actively, Healthily, Vigorously

BY **CLEMENT G. MARTIN**, M. D.
Former Medical Director
CONTINENTAL CASUALTY COMPANY

With a Foreword by Edward R.
Annis, M. D., President of the
American Medical Association

FREDERICK FELL INC.
NEW YORK 16, N. Y.

Manufactured in the United States of America

Library of Congress Catalog Card No. 63-14284

Published simultaneously in Canada by
George McLeod, Ltd., 73 Bathurst St., Toronto, Ont.

"To those who have shown me the art of living I dedicate this study of the science of living."

FOREWORD

The medical profession, throughout time, has made discoveries and strides of progress that have literally altered
the courses of whole civilizations. Remarkable as this might
seem, it is, perhaps, even more remarkable to know that
the medical profession has scored its most startling and
significant breakthroughs just within the last 100 years
or so.

The veritable parade of monumental discoveries and de-
velopments in the health fields was made possible largely
through an impetus found only in the atmosphere of free
and private enterprise, and it is really this that has provided
our present day civilization with the finest fruits of a Golden
Age of Medicine.

Certainly not the least important of medical science's more
recent contributions is the gift of longevity. Medical re-
searchers, to now, have already discovered many of nature's
secrets of life, and these findings have enabled us to prolong
our days on earth in active, good health.

A child who is born today can expect to live seven years
longer than one born just 20 years ago; and a person who
is 70 years of age today has already lived twice as long as
the average American at the time of our Revolution, for the

life expectancy at that time was only 35 years! And this, many medical authorities believe, represents our scratching only at the surface of the problem.

Clement Martin, a doctor of medicine and an author, is one authority who believes just that. Writing in clear, entertaining, and understandable language in "How To Live To Be 100," he sees no reason why human beings should not, even on the basis of medical data we possess today, live to attain five score or more years of life. His book is a practical treatise on how to do this.

"How To Live To Be 100" is an optimistic book when examined by the cold stare of the questioning scientist. Nevertheless it emphasizes the proper areas and approach to keeping healthy and fit—nutrition, periodic medical care, dental services, choice of satisfying work endeavor, healthy play and recreation, rest, exercise, and relaxation. And it emphasizes what the American medical profession has long maintained—that the well being of a person just as the quality of medicine itself, is the responsibility not of a community or a government agency but of each individual himself. This point is well worth remembering.

Author Martin cannot guarantee that his readers will actually live to be 100; only that you should live longer, healthier, and more enjoyably if you follow his advice.

Edward R. Annis, M.D.
President
American Medical Association
Chicago, Illinois

CONTENTS

PART 3

Longevity and Common Sense

a. CAUSES OF DEATH IN PROFESSIONAL MEN
b. HEART ATTACKS DON'T WAIT FOR OLD AGE
c. BLOOD PRESSURE AND LIFE EXPECTANCY
d. POSSIBILITIES OF LIFE EXPECTANCY
e. THE AMAZING STORY OF MR. MARATHON

INTRODUCTION

Your health is the most valuable investment you own.

Stocks, bonds, cash and other physical possessions are changeable and expendable. But your health is an asset that you must conserve in order to enjoy anything else in life. Therefore, it is vital for you to realize this fact:

You can live to one hundred healthy, productive years, simply by applying the knowledge doctors now have about longevity.

In fact, one hundred and twenty-five years of activity and vitality should be the attainable goal for mankind. All other mammals live for five times the number of years it takes them to reach maturity. Man reaches his skeletal maturity about the age of twenty-six.[1] This indicates one hundred years of productive life as a reasonable goal for all of us.

Yet life expectancy today is only sixty-eight for men, and seventy-three for women. Why? Chiefly because of these two factors:

1) Over half the deaths among adults today are caused by the "disease of civilization"—arteriosclerosis. Most of these deaths can be prevented.[2] The simple fitness program presented in this book will show you how.

2) Nearly another one-quarter of the deaths occurring after thirty-five are caused by cancer. This statistic can be

cut to less than one-half [3] by means of health audit exams, such as the example given later in this book.

As citizens of a well-informed country, we are already aware that obesity is a great threat to a long life. But we have failed to take full advantage of the great benefits of regular physical activity. In fact, the prime reason for the great number of deaths occurring in the early autumn of life is the lack of such intelligently-supervised physical effort.

Until today, we have literally been killing ourselves with good living. We did not realize that simply by making a few changes, we could live equally as well—and gain thirty to forty healthy, active vigorous years doing it.

Yes, one hundred years is our goal. But we cannot have them by demanding them from someone. We must earn these extra years. We must earn our life and strength just as we earn our income—personally.

The knowledge that can be used for this great increase in both age and vitality is before you in this book. It is not hard to understand. It is not hard to apply. It requires only a little effort—mental, physical, habitual. But the decision to make this effort must come from you, after reading and digesting this book.

Here, then, is a practical, realistic program for the full use of a long and healthy life. It can be applied by any man or woman of any age from seventeen to seventy, who can pass the simple test described in Chapter 5.

If you wish not only to live longer, but to enjoy every year of your life, you start here.

REFERENCES CITED IN THIS CHAPTER

1. Raab, W. Dr., *Annals of Internal Medicine* 54:6, 1961.
2. Bortz, E. L., M.D., *Encyclopedia Brittanica, Book of the Year,* 1961.
3. Portes, Caeser, M.D., in a personal communication to the author.

HOW TO LIVE TO BE 100

Part One

What This Book Can Do For You—A Healthy, Active, Vigorous Life Till the Age of One Hundred

Part One

Chapter One

YOUR TRUE LIFE EXPECTANCY—HOW LONG SHOULD YOU REALLY BE ABLE TO LIVE

Your life span has been investigated for many years. For example, two centuries ago the French scientist Buffon calculated that the natural life span of a man was 125 to 150 years. He reasoned in this way:

All other mammals live to five times the number of years it takes their skeleton to mature. A dog's skeleton matures at three; their normal life is fifteen to sixteen years. Man's skeleton matures at twenty-five to twenty-eight years of age—so 125 years or better are his calculated days.

ACTIVE LIVES AT 120

People are living to these ages with vigor and virility today in at least two parts of the world. Many of us know of the story of Hunza, in the Himalayas. These people are living active lives at 120 and more. Men beget children when they are in their nineties. Studies of these people show that, out of economic necessity, they do many of the things research has shown are needed for longevity.

In addition, in Rajshapur, India, many of its citizens also live to advanced years in excellent health—well over a hundred. Their mode of life also causes practice of the same principles of good health that we all should adopt.

GREAT GAINS IN LONGEVITY ALREADY

Such principles of good health have already tripled our average life spans, as the following quotation shows:

"From studies of skeletal remains, it has been estimated that the average length of life in the early Iron and Bronze Age was about 18 years.

"The indications provided from certain burial inscriptions in Ancient Rome are not much better, the average for that period being about 22 years.

"Although at a higher level of about 33 years there was apparently little change in the average length of life in the Western world from the Middle Ages until the time of our Revolution.

"Over these centuries, during which the average length of life may have been anywhere from 30 to 35 years, there was an utter lack of sanitation and little knowledge of preventive medicine. Progress in these directions had to wait until the dawn of the agricultural and industrial revolution.

"By the middle of the last century the average length of life rose to about 40 years and it took fully one-half century to raise this average to 49 years in the United States.

"However, during the next half-century, the average length of life in our country rose by nearly 20 years, to a level of 68.6 years in 1952.

"This, then, is the measure of the effect of modern medicine and of advances in public health upon longevity.

OLD KILLERS CONQUERED

"This past half-century has been one of extraordinary reductions in mortality, but the gains have come primarily from the control of infection.

". . . contrast the situation in the United States in 1900 and 1954. At the earlier date, the list of causes of death was headed by three infectious conditions; pneumonia and influenza with a death rate of 202 per 100,000; tuberculosis with a rate of 194; and diarrhea and enteritis with 143. Diphtheria ranked among the first 10 causes of death with a rate of 40 per 100,000. These few infectious conditions alone accounted for one-third of all deaths in the United States in 1900.

"On the other hand, by 1954 the death rate from pneumonia and influenza had been reduced to about one-eighth the level at the beginning of the century, and these conditions rank only sixth among the causes of death. Tuberculosis no longer ranks among the first 10 causes, while diarrhea, enteritis and diphtheria are among the very minor ones.

"In fact, there has been a reversal of the significance of the important causes of death. The cardiovascular conditions —diseases of the heart, cerebral hemorrhage and nephritis —and cancer are now in the forefront.

"*In other words, there has been a shift from the diseases of infancy, childhood and early life to the conditions typical of mid-life and old age . . .*" (Italics mine) [1]

NEW VICTORIES TO BE WON

But as the story of the Hunza shows us, we are only half-way towards our goal. Our job today is to take this average American life expectancy of 68 years, and double it—or nearly double it—again.

To do this, we must first examine the great killers of our adult lives—the diseases which stand in the way of our living healthy, active lives till one hundred.

REFERENCE CITED IN THIS CHAPTER

1. *The Relation of Longevity to Life Insurance Selection,* Chapter 13, by Louis Dublin, Ph.D.—from Life Insurance and Medicine, Edited by Harry E. Ungerleider, M.D., F.A.C.P. and Richard Gubner, M.D., F.A.C.P.

Chapter Two

WHY ARE WE BEING DEPRIVED OF A LONGER LIFE?

What prevents us from attaining this goal of 100, 115, or 125 years? We can find many of the answers to this question by looking at the two diseases that cause most of the deaths of middle age.

1) *The Great Killer of Our Times*

Prime killer in adult life is arteriosclerosis, accounting for better than 55% of all deaths, registered at all ages.

The deaths caused by arteriosclerosis are those that are attributed to hardening of the arteries. Among them are heart attacks, strokes and senility.

Heart attacks alone account for nearly half the total deaths due to hardening of the arteries. These heart attacks are the greatest single cause of our shortened life span. Men, and to an ever-increasing extent, women also, die from coronary heart disease in their forties, fifties and early sixties.

Strokes are the greatest fear of the aged. Death is not always the immediate result of a stroke; disability is the far more frequent occurrence. Long periods of invalidism—

ranging from an inability to use a hand or leg, up to states so severe as to leave the afflicted person no more than a vegetable—are the results of this brain damage from arteriosclerosis.

Senility is also most often caused by the hardening of the arteries in our brains. Attacking this problem is a matter of personal concern for us all, requiring not only national, but individual effort.

2) Cancer Deaths Can Be Cut in Half

Cancer accounts for about 20% of the deaths in the U.S. today. This figure could be reduced to less than half its present toll if periodic cancer detection examinations were a national habit, rather than the exceptional effort of a few that they are now.

Periodic health examinations will also place us in the hands of a doctor for many other diseases that only he can detect in the early, most curable stages.

Let's Look at the Figures

The accompanying charts dramatically show the increased death rates caused by just one of these killers—hardening of the arteries. Of great importance in studying these charts are these two facts:

1) Notice the tremendous difference in death rates between professions. The more successful the man, the more inactive his life, and the greater chance he has of dying young.

2) And, even more important, coronary disease can be avoided by the methods described in this book. These tragedies do not have to take place at all! The rest of this book is devoted to preventing them.

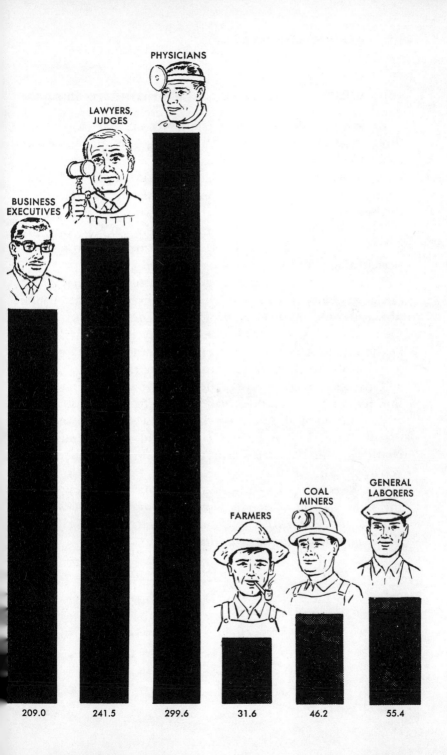

BUSINESS
EXECUTIVES

LAWYERS,
JUDGES

PHYSICIANS

FARMERS

COAL
MINERS

GENERAL
LABORERS

209.0   241.5   299.6   31.6   46.2   55.4

HIGH EARNING GROUPS ARE HIGH DEATH RATE GROUPS

In this and the following chart we see, too clearly, the threat that the sedentary—high earning—occupations make against our lives.

We feel that we should raise our children to be "something," and we do our best to place them, and ourselves, in these occupations that kill through sitting.

These deaths represent more than personal loss; they are a drain on the economy of the country. Training, experience and skills are lost—irrecoverably.

A farmer can be nearly as good a farmer at thirty as he can be at eighty. This is not true of the executives, attorneys, physicians and most other professional men. At thirty these men are still learning their tasks; at forty they are first really beginning to know about their jobs; and the years from fifty on are their years of greatest importance.

This loss to themselves, their families and their community is not only unfortunate; it is a needless waste.

Prevention of this loss of the highly skilled is the aim of this book. We, as individuals, should want to meet the challenge the Russians have thrown down by their preventive health maintenance.

The facts are clear—The more sedentary the occupation, the more dangerous it is! *Three and one half times more deaths, from hardening of the arteries, occur among professional men than among unskilled laborers.*

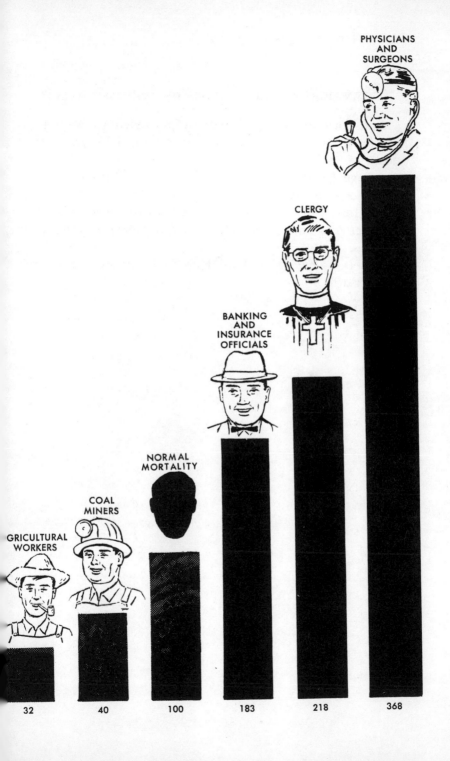

PHYSICIANS
AND
SURGEONS

CLERGY

BANKING
AND
INSURANCE
OFFICIALS

NORMAL
MORTALITY

COAL
MINERS

GRICULTURAL
WORKERS

32   40   100   183   218   368

EVEN MORE APPALLING COSTS OF "TOO-EASY LIVING"

And not only does our civilized and sedentary way of living cause us to die too early, but it also makes invalids of many of us before death.

At age 55 about ten per cent of any civilized country's work force is on disability pensions. Almost all of these early, forced retirements are the consequences of strokes, heart attacks and other results of hard arteries and flabby muscles.

Something had to be done. Here's what it was—and here's what it did!

Chapter Three

WHAT RESULTS CAN YOU EXPECT? HOW TO ADD UP TO FORTY VIGOROUS YEARS TO YOUR LIFE!

These facts state the problem clearly. Without question, something should be done about exercise and diet for our high earning, high-living and high death-rate population.

WHAT EUROPE IS DOING

This unnecessary human wastage has caused many European countries to ask themselves what can be done to stop it. What mass rehabilitation programs can be instituted to avoid these losses?

Since physical inactivity is the cause of this invalidism and death, planned exercise programs seem to be the answer.

The first of these exercise programs was begun in the Bavarian mountains: the "Ohlstadter Kur" initiated in 1953 by Beckmann. This has been a model for similar exercise programs in other parts of Germany, Austria, Greece, Holland and Israel, Norway and Yugoslavia.

THE SOVIET ANSWER

A great deal of work of a similar nature is being done in the U.S.S.R. Each year five million Soviet citizens are given a month in the country. During this time they are given physical fitness training, and knowledge on diet and medical self-help. The Russians state that this will be a method of increasing life span, and "also beating capitalism in the field of economy." [1]

EXERCISE BREAKS INSTEAD OF COFFEE BREAKS

In Sweden and in many other continental countries the "coffee break" of our country is replaced by exercise breaks for ten to twenty minutes.

Each group within the office or factory does planned physical activity under the leadership of their supervisor, a person who has been especially trained for this program.

This is an activity pattern we all must learn to avoid waste of muscles and waste of life that our sedentary civilization is producing in us.

LET'S LOOK AT THE FIGURES AGAIN

But, if something is done about adding exercise and even diet, what sort of results can be anticipated?

The continental rehabilitation camps have not been in existence long enough to show much in the way of statistics and, of course, the statistics they do present are on the basis of an intensive four- to six-week program. However, the following facts have already become apparent:

BETTER GENERAL HEALTH

Between 1957 and 1959, 86.3% participants in one of the reconditioning centers remained free of illness although the same individuals had been repeatedly ill before that period.[2]

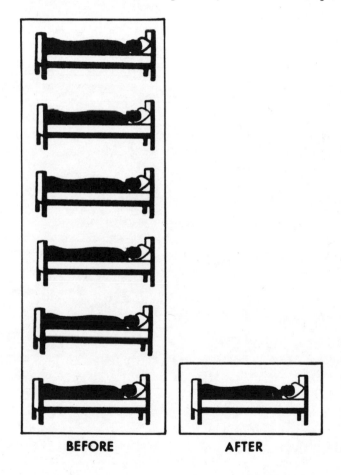

BEFORE   **AFTER**

FAR LESS HEART ATTACKS

The Russians state that only one cardiovascular death in the USSR occurs for every 2.38 such deaths in the United States.[3]

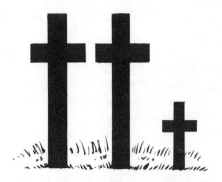

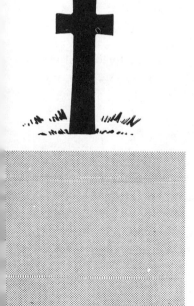

USSR

USA

Important work in the United States has been done by Mr. W. V. Cumler of the Central Branch of the Cleveland YMCA. The following chart shows the results on reducing diastolic blood pressures by means of a model program of calisthenics and running activities.[4]

Let us look at each of these men in turn, and see how many years of life expectancy they gained by following this program for a few months.

58 YEARS ADDED TO LIFE EXPECTANCY OF THESE FOUR MEN, through these simple methods in a few short months.

SUBJECT A

Pulse too rapid, blood pressure too high. On the surface this man's problems might not seem great. Yet his blood pressure showed he had only one-half the normal life expectancy for his age.

In two months of an exercise program he had improved to a normal blood pressure, and his life expectancy had gained thirteen years.

SUBJECT B

A younger man with really bad blood pressure. He had less than a third of normal life expectancy; certainly he was not someone whom the insurance companies were going to want on their books.

At the end of his fourth month of exercise he had a more efficient pulse; and much better chances for long life—about 18 years more.

EXTENSION OF LIFE EXPECTANCY

Subject	Test Number	After Months of Exercise	Pulse Rate	Blood Pressure	Age	Life Expectancy in Years	
						Before	After
A	1		112	138/102	45	12	25
	2	2	88	142/85			
B	1		94	190/106	44	7	25
	2	4	68	145/79			
C	1		84	168/114	43	9	29
	2	3	70	122/83			
D	1		93	168/104	61	7	14
	2	20	44	127/68			

Fifty-eight years expectancy were added to these four men.

SUBJECT C

The blood pressure reading shown on this man's chart was far from the highest that he had; it represented instead the lowest that he was able to attain by using certain high-blood-pressure medicines.

When he started the fitness program, his physician reminded him of the importance of keeping his nurse informed of his general health, in order to make certain his medications remained at a proper level.

But these words fell on deaf ears! At some time during the second month of activity, he felt so fine he decided to quit taking the medication!

In spite of this, his test at the end of the third month showed a normal blood pressure—with a truly tremendous increase in life expectancy amounting to twenty extra years.

SUBJECT D

This case proves that you don't have to be young to give your heart and arteries the benefits of regular exercise. This individual shows a change from the first test to the second that is most dramatic.

Pulse and both phases of blood pressure have gone from the too-frequently-seen findings of neglected middle age to those that many an Olympic athlete maintains. Life expectancy has doubled.

A PERSONAL NOTE

All life expectancies shown above are valid statistical assumptions based on the best medical information currently available. However, the author does not believe that they truly reflect the great improvement in life expectancy that these individuals will enjoy. The increase should amount to many years more than these figures indicate.

REFERENCES CITED IN THIS CHAPTER

1. Foreign Letters JAMA 175:65, 1961.
2. Raab, W., M.D. *Annals of Internal Medicine* 54:6, 1961.
3. Carter, C., Carter, D., Cancer, Smoking, Heart Disease, Drinking in our Two-World System Today. Northern Book House, Toronto, 1958.
4. Cumler, W. V. Physical Fitness Program for Men Y.M.C.A. Central Branch, Cleveland, Ohio.

Chapter Four

FURTHER REWARDS OF FITNESS

"The possession of physical strength, agility and endurance may enable the individual to survive, while the lack of fitness may spell catastrophe." [1]

These words express the thoughtful opinion of the American Medical Association and the American Association for Health, Physical Education and Recreation on the prime value of fitness—*survival*.

But what of its other values? What good is it to live to be a hundred unless you have the health, strength, vitality, vigor—yes even virility, that make your later years worthwhile! Can fitness give you all these in addition to mere longevity?

The answer most emphatically is YES! Here are just a few of the subsidiary benefits you can expect from this fitness program—benefits that will begin in a few short days, and continue for decades of enjoyable living.

A STRONGER HEART AND LUNGS

The statement of the doctors and physical educators quoted above does not stop at mere comments concerning the relation of fitness and long life. Prolonged inactivity, they say, is marked by a decline in the efficiency of both our hearts and our lungs. This is the same story that the rest of life teaches us: no resting on the oars. You must either swim upstream, or drift downstream to disaster.

This joint statement of the A. M. A. goes on to tell us that as we engage in a fitness program, our heart and circulatory system will be trained to become far more efficient. This efficiency will be demonstrated in more economical pumping action of the heart, throughout the entire body. And not only will our heart and blood vessels work better—our lungs will also increase in efficiency.

BETTER CIRCULATION

Physical fitness won't grow hair for the bald headed, but it will help to maintain what hair you have through better circulation—and perhaps through the increased attention you give your entire body.

Your blood vessels, principally your arteries, are going to get bigger and better. Various studies have shown that the arteries of physically active people are up to four or five times larger than the arteries of the sitters. At least as important is the equally well demonstrated fact that you will grow new blood vessels, and provide your body with a better circulation than it originally had.[2]

GREATER REGULARITY

With your improved posture and strength the internal organs of your body will function with greater regularity.

Your body was constructed with a correct place for every organ in it. But years of faulty posture have pushed and pulled many people's internal architecture into new, surrealistic arrangements that don't work well. The commonest symptom of this displacement is that of bowel upsets. In women, furthermore, menstrual disorders also occur.

Experimental evidence has shown that a program of fitness reduces these functional disorders that are so common today. Bowel upsets, constipation and menstrual disorders all have been shown to have benefitted from a regular program of exercise. What a far cry these facts are from our folk-lore!

BETTER APPEARANCE

Are you a real man? Are you a real woman? With true physical health you will both look and act the part.

Look at most people in the street to see what I mean. They don't walk, they slouch along. They don't stand, they lean—or tilt. They don't have good skin. At a distance it is often impossible to guess whether a male or female is coming down the road toward you!

I can promise you this. As you gain the strength and endurance you need for good health, you will find that people suddenly notice *you*. Not your clothing, your mannerisms or some other decoration that you carry with you— they see *you*. A vital human being to be admired and imitated.

GREATER VITALITY

We all wish to get ahead. How many of us are really content to sacrifice our chances of personal, social and business success to the constant threat of poor health?

Action, participation and recognition are what we all want. As we develop our bodies, we will find our energies more responsive and more dependable—and our goals suddenly attainable.

A GLOWING COMPLEXION

Your skin will acquire a glow previously unknown. This comes from a new exposure to elements from this program.

The use your skin gets in exercise and in outdoor activities acts as a far finer balm than any to be found on the cosmetic shelves.

Of course, this is not to be interpreted as meaning that you should go too far in exposing your skin to fresh air and sunshine. A little of anything is good, too much is always bad.

Sitting on the beach is neither a form of exercise, nor a good hobby for those who wish to have a youthful skin in the last years. White skin ages with sunlight—black, red and brown skin is of much better quality; it does not age in the sunlight.

IMPROVED MENTAL POWERS

These are not the only benefits of a sound, fit body. Your mental stamina and resilience will improve in direct proportion to the attainment of your goals of fitness.

A sound mind in a sound body is a most unfortunate way of expressing this truth. We are not a person made up of parts; each of us is an organic unit. We think, feel and reason with the section of this unit called the brain. It needs a good supply of blood and other nourishment to carry out its functions. Insure that supply and it will give you performance and endurance that may amaze you.

GREATER SEXUAL VIGOR

Those who are fit already know, apparently as a delightful secret, that fitness will greatly improve sexual vigor.

Let me repeat this fact. Those peoples of the Earth today who attain ages beyond a hundred also apparently enjoy sexual activity into their last decades. Men have fathered children when they were ninety years of age. Can there be any greater proof of over-all physical vigor?

On the other hand sexual activity, since it involves great muscular work, can be a disastrous overload for one out of condition. Certainly some heart attacks are related to the sudden efforts of love making.

BETTER MEMORIES AS WE GROW OLDER

The too frequent mental lapses of the aged are often due to insufficient circulation of blood through their brain. Such lapses may appear to be overnight disasters, but they rarely are. Usually a lack of circulation has been caused by years of continuous sitting, by over eating, and by other habits of a lifetime devoted to unfitness.

If you like the way you can think today, and if you want to retain it for decades to come, reflect—then act—to keep fit.

MORE FUN, MORE ENERGY. MORE PEP— RIGHT UP PAST NINETY!

Last of all, with all these benefits coming to you through a simple, moderate change in your way of doing things, your disposition must improve—it has no choice.

"Rush, rush—time is running out," can sound quite real if you look at the mortality tables and hope for average luck.

But that same cry of woe loses much of its urgency when you look at it from the perspective of a life only half lived at fifty; with the best—freedom, health and wisdom—yet to be savored after ninety.

REFERENCES CITED IN THIS CHAPTER

1. J. A. M. A. April 5, 1958.
2. Eckstein, R. W. Circulation Research 5, 230, 1957.

Part Two

Your Personal Fitness Program

Chapter Five

HOW FIT—OR UNFIT—ARE YOU TODAY?
TRY THESE SIMPLE TESTS

How fit are you today? How much do you need to improve to gain the maximum longevity? And how fast will you improve?

Some type of testing is needed to know where we stand today, and how we're doing as we improve.

A QUICK FITNESS QUIZ

Lists of the various symptoms that unfitness causes in all of us could be made into a fair-sized book. Right now, to get a quick idea of your present state of fitness, check yourself with the few questions here:

1. Are you "worn out" long before bedtime?
2. Do your feet hurt day after day?
3. Is your back a source of annoyance and pain?
4. Do you mind standing when you have to wait for a moment, or do you immediately try to find a place to lean or sit?

5. If you have to run for a train or cab, are you huffing and puffing for half an hour? Or do you shudder at the very thought?

6. Do you think it would be possible for you to run up a flight of stairs today without strain?

7. Are you bothered with stomach and bowel upsets?

8. Do you have frequent headaches?

9. Do you bounce out of bed in the morning—or crawl out?

10. Do you have trouble relaxing?

11. Do you have trouble sleeping soundly at night?

12. Do you suffer from frequent, unexplained tensions and a feeling of restlessness?

In other words, *are you really satisfied with your present physical condition?*

And are you going to do anything about that condition? If your answer is Yes, then here's the information you need!

WHAT SHALL WE MEASURE?

Before we go into actual physical tests themselves, let's state what it is we want to know from them.

Strength, agility and endurance are all part of physical fitness. To live to be a hundred, or a hundred ten or a hundred twenty, we must have all three.

However, strength we will have in sufficient amounts if we stay in training at all. Strength testing, then, can be largely eliminated from our fitness tests. Though, of course, if you find yourself at an amusement park next to a grip tester, go ahead, put in your dime and test your strength— it's fun. But there is no need to buy one of these dynamometers and bring it home; wait until you're back at the park next year.

Agility also is subject to testing, but none of these agility tests are easy to give or to interpret. Sufficient agility also will be gained, and even checked by, endurance training.

YOUR MAIN GOAL IS ENDURANCE

Endurance testing should be continued over long periods of time—for it is such endurance tests that reveal to us the true measure of our body's ability to withstand strain.

This type of testing can also, in fact, constitute training in itself, since it gives us a definite, strenuous work load to perform over a short period of time. No expensive or unusual gadgets are needed for the two endurance tests listed here. But the presence of an objective observer can be of great assistance in making sure the test is done correctly.

1) THE SIMPLE PULSE RATE TEST

Years ago life insurance companies found that measuring the pulse rate before and after exercise was a good, quick, reliable method of estimating health in its relation to longevity. Over the years this type of testing has been the object of much research and improvement. Here's how it now goes:

(1) First, take your pulse while sitting at rest.

(2) Then hop fifty times, twenty-five hops on each foot.

(3) Take your pulse immediately after the last hop.

(4) Sit for two minutes, then take your pulse again.

While you are hopping, an experienced observer could tell a great deal about your health simply by watching you; in fact, he could actually guess the pulse rate he will find at the end of the exercise.

For example, in insurance examinations, sometimes a young, lean prospect literally leaps through the hops, is done in no time, and has increased his pulse rate only slightly.

The next examination may give the examiner a humorous contrast as some heavy, flabby man of importance does the soft shoe shuffle for fifty times—puffing wildly at the end of his greatest activity in ages.

THE HEALTHY INDIVIDUAL SHOWS UP THIS WAY

In any case, a normal pulse at rest—before the test—should be somewhere in between sixty and eighty-five beats per minute. Highly trained athletes may have a pulse lower than sixty; down to fifty or forty-eight is frequent. In the average person, though, a pulse as slow as that is more apt to indicate a heart problem than good physical condition.

After the test, an increase of the pulse up to an extra fifty beats per minute is considered satisfactory. Satisfactory in this instance means having what is now considered "normal" life expectancy. It is not really satisfactory for those of us who want to live out many years beyond the "averages" in vitality. We should strive to have an increase of no more than an extra twenty beats per minute.

After the two-minute rest period, your pulse should have slowed down to about the rate first observed. Five or ten beats one way or the other are about the proper limits.

To repeat before the test, your pulse rate should be 60 to 85 beats per minute. Immediately after the test, it should have increased to no more than 110 to 118 beats per minute, and preferably to only 90 to 100 beats per minute. After a two-minute rest, it should have returned to within 5 or 10 beats of your normal.

The healthier subject will usually show an actual reduction in his pulse rate after exercise. The untrained, dangerously out of condition man is the one who can't get his pulse rate down to even ten beats of its original rate.

The accompanying chart gives you the needed information to be checked in this examination.

Chart No. 1

PULSE RATE:	NORMAL RESULTS:
Resting	60 to 85
Fifty hops	90 to 140
Two minutes rest	60 to 95

HOW TO FIND A PULSE

It is better to have someone else take your pulse, if possible. Not only will the examination be more accurate at rest this way; but a lot more meaningful after the exercise —when huffing, puffing and body tremors may really cause confusion if you take your own pulse.

If you have difficulty knowing how to take a pulse, a few words may help you, or your associate, in discovering where it is, and what messages it is sending.

Most people have their pulse beat located on the side of the wrist near the thumb. (*See Illustration*) In some individuals, however, it may be located on the top of the wrist or on the side near the little finger.

In feeling for the pulse, never use your thumb, since it has its own pulse, and you will find these beats confusing and adding to the pulse rate at the wrist.

Sometimes no one can find a pulse at the wrist. Either the artery lies too deep to give a perceptible impulse, or the artery has spread out into several small branches. If this is the case, the best advice is to look for a good pulse elsewhere.

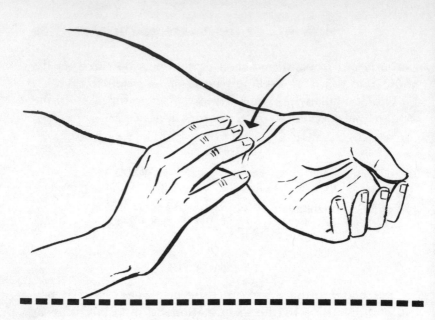

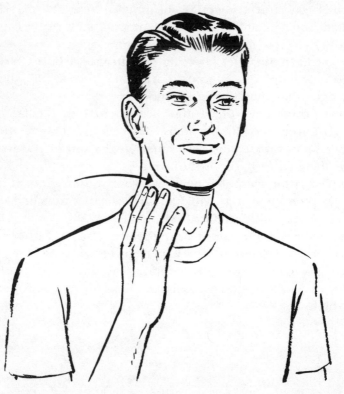

The neck is the best place to find a pulse in a fairly constant location. Place your three fingers together on your neck at a position midway between a line drawn down from the ear and center of the neck. You will undoubtedly feel some sort of pulsation. Slowly, and without too much pressure, move your fingers from this point either to the center of the neck, or back to the ear. (See Illustration).

Exploring in this manner will quickly show you where the strongest point of pulsation occurs. Once you have found the pulse in your own neck you will be able to find it readily in another's.

HOW TO READ THE PULSE'S MESSAGE

Finding the pulse can give us a sense of satisfaction, but if we are to profit from this discovery, we should then learn a few of its signs.

A healthy pulse has a good bounce and will keep on with its regular rhythm even as it is put under moderate finger pressure. If you find a pulse that seems more like a little pipe, hard and lumpy, you are dealing with a hard artery.

Although this is not the same type of hard artery associated with heart failure, it is a sufficient warning to stop further pulse testing and seek medical attention. This does not mean you should run to the emergency room—but you should call and make an appointment in the next week or so. It took years for the artery to get this hard, and medical help will be needed for any fitness schedule.

The pulse also may seem small. Physicians usually use the term, thready. As you might suspect, such an unusually small pulse represents a heart that is not pumping a full, adequate supply of blood to the body. Once again, go to your doctor and get his advice.

Any pulse that is not giving a regular rhythmic beat is also to be suspected. Fortunately irregular pulses are rare. But if you find a rate that does not read out like 1-1-1-1 you have a problem. Abnormal pulses may read: 1—1,2-1,1,1—— 1,2, or 1,1,1,—1.

However, if your pulse is normal, and you know of no other disease, then it is safe to go ahead with the remainder of the test.

EFFECT OF THE TEST ON YOUR PULSE

This type of test is an excellent place for most of us to start. It can serve as a speedy reassurance for those in fair to good condition, and as a real warning to those too far out of condition.

If you *can't* pass this test, as shown above, your exercise program must start out more slowly than would otherwise be advisable.

Too many of today's successful men and women—irreplaceable leaders in the community—have gained their positions of prominence through hard mental work and self-control. If these same people leap with full force into an exercise program, they will misinterpret the term "vigorous" to their own disadvantage. Knowing from previous experience vigor in mental activities, they may expect their bodies to be capable of as much strain as their mentalities.

Therefore, you should adopt your exercise program to the results of this test in this way:

Even if the resting pulse is over 85, but under 95, it is still safe to go ahead with the test.

However, if any signs of strain, shortness of breath, chest discomfort or dizziness appear during the hops, stop immediately and check pulse. As long as it remains below 150 there is no need for concern. This indicates, usually, too much weight and too little physical reserve. In the *specific exercises* to follow, rope skipping should be avoided until this test can be passed, and the walking program should be restricted to a maximum of fast walking—no trotting.

If, however, the resting pulse does not return to five or ten points within the two-minute interval, keep on checking it at two-minute intervals. If it has returned to normal by four minutes there is no need for alarm, but the need of a fitness program is even more definite. However, at six minutes the pulse rate had better be down to normal limits if you wish to carry out any plans that take more than pushing a button to do. If not, consult your doctor.

However, though this pulse test is a good benchmark—it will not do to show real fitness—nor can it serve to show one's progress in an objective, meaningful manner. For those objectives, we must turn to—

2) THE 17-INCH BENCH-STEP TEST

The test chosen to help us in this progress objective is the one utilized in the President's booklet on *Adult Fitness*. This is a real endurance test. Even if you have breezed through the first test, don't expect to be a star in this test right off.

This second test is known as the Seventeen-Inch Bench-Step Test. It has been extensively checked and standardized by the Air Force at Randolph Field. It can be done with a minimum of equipment and will give accurate results.

A bench that measures exactly seventeen inches in height need not be purchased—nearly any sturdy chair in the house can be put into service. Its basic requirement is that of stability and strength; for in doing the test, this chair or bench is going to be carrying all your weight. If you have a good metal dinette chair, it will probably be ideal.

Also, its height does not have to be an exact seventeen inches to get reasonably accurate results in your tests. Any height between fifteen and eighteen inches will serve sufficiently well.

And since the technique of the test demands that you step up on the chair first with one foot, then with the other, your own height should have some consideration in selecting a proper height surface for stepping. A woman five feet tall is going to work very hard stepping up seventeen inches, and a six foot six man may not be working hard enough by only raising himself up the same seventeen inches.

HERE'S HOW YOU DO THIS TEST

To get the best results, this test should be done two or three hours after a meal, and only when you are feeling reasonably well. A slight cold or even a mild headache will just get worse during the test and fail to give a correct estimate of your fitness.

You don't need a new outfit of gym clothes, of course, but clothing should be kept at a minimum, and your pockets should be empty. Whether or not you have shoes on does not make a great deal of difference, but most people find it easiest to do the exam barefooted.

It makes no difference which foot you begin the test with, but for the purpose of description we will follow the ancient tradition and start with the left foot. Here we go:

Take, or have someone else take your pulse. Stand next to the chair.

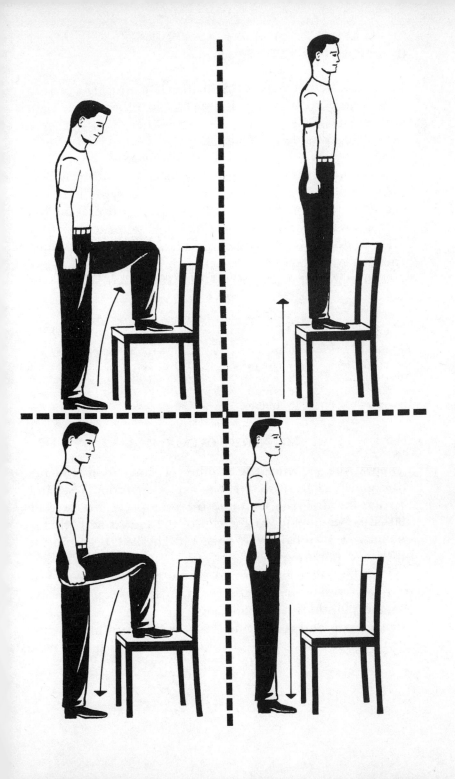

(1) Raise your left foot up on the chair quickly.

(2) Raise your body up on the chair by placing your right foot on the chair.

(3) Bring your left foot down.

(4) And then bring your right foot down.

As you do this, if you can find sufficient breath, count 1, 2, 3, 4 in sequence with the four different steps. This will give you a little timing and rhythm, and it will prevent you from slowing down in going through this set of tests.

Try to do this four count exercise at a rate of thirty times a minute. And always go through each step in sequence—we are examining for endurance, not for strength.

	Stepping Time	Pulse Rates	
		Men	Women
Beginning	30 seconds	100 or less	110 or less
Intermediate	1 minute	100 or less	110 or less
Advanced	2 minutes	100 or less	110 or less
Energetic	3 minutes	140 or less	150 or less
Dynamic	5 minutes	150 or less	160 or less

NO NEED TO OVER-DO IT

Repeat the sequence the number of times shown on the chart above: Start with the beginner's 30-second test, and increase the time you continue till your pulse rate exceeds 100 beats per minute. At the end of the test sit and rest for one minute, then have your pulse rate checked, beginning at the second minute of rest.

Don't be a hero in trying to go too fast too soon. If you try to do more of the test than your pulse says you are ready for, the punishment is inglorious.

Somewhere during the time your legs will quit and without them the nearest part of your anatomy will be the next in line to bear your weight. Usually well padded, your derriere will protect you from grave injury; but the mental blow is nearly insufferable as you find it necessary to crawl to a corner to nurse your injury.

However, if you are sincere in keeping at this program, good results are going to be seen in a month and dramatic ones in two months.

And, above all, don't be discouraged by your performance in comparison to the ideal last two sections of this test. These final two sections may never be within your range of accomplishment. They are performance standards that Olympic athletes and astronauts must make. But the closer you come to attaining this degree of fitness, the more you are doing to assure yourself of the healthy added years you want.

Chapter Six

YOUR NEW OUTLOOK ON LIFE

Now to get started on a healthier, more enjoyable, longer life. To do this, we simply alter a few of our present habits.

Most of us have developed these present habits by accident—not by thought. In the good old days before Cro-Magnon Man, this kind of accidental formation of habits was fine. Since one had to do strenuous work to eat, it did permit the most fit to survive.

But since that time, the evolution of man has been progressively one of less body and more mind. This evolution is going on at a startling pace today. The demands on our bodies have become far less strenuous and the demands on our minds far greater than ever in the past.

For example, in 1860 thirty per cent of the energy provided in the United States for building, logging and all other industries was supplied by muscle power. Today, less than one per cent of all the energy used in the United States is derived from man's muscles.

STRONGER BODY—STRONGER MIND

We must deliberately take care of our body if our body —and our brain—are to function well. This has been dramatically shown in studies of undergraduates at West Point. Those that entered in good physical condition had the smallest number of emotional upsets and maintained the best average grades. Those who just skimmed through on their fitness testing did poorly in their academic work and had a very high incidence of nervous breakdowns.

RESULTS SHOW QUICKLY

Redoing our habits is going to take some effort. How much effort depends largely on what our present habits are. But no matter how much remodeling is required, no one needs a great deal of time to achieve his goals. By the end of a few short months, all of us should be comfortably along toward a life of health, vigor and fitness.

None of these changes are totally different from what we do now. They are more or less the addition and subtraction of a few habits in our total scheme of living. I do not propose, for example, to ban smoking, drinking, or any of the minor civilized vices. Dr. Gallup has shown that those who live longest are those who enjoy life. It is the purpose of this book to make your life more enjoyable, more vital, and precisely as long as it should be.

EXERCISE FOR LONG LIFE

The two major changes needed in most of our lives are exercise and diet.

The exercise we need does not have to be lengthy, nor does it require the purchase of a single unit of expensive equipment. Three half-hours a week devoted to pleasant physical activities will bring us to prime physical fitness and keep us in top shape.

The benefits of such a program can be evaluated by its effect on only one symptom of life expectancy—blood pressure. Test after test has shown that even as little as a few months of this type of fitness activity increases the life span through dramatically reducing high blood pressure.

If you now have high blood pressure of this type—hypertension—you most certainly should consult your physician before beginning this exercise program. But you will find that this high blood pressure is never going to stop you from such a fitness program. It will only slow down your entrance into the most vigorous forms of it.

DIET FOR LONG LIFE

Diet-needs must change for most of us if we are to avoid the early deaths of these times.

Lumberjacks and construction workers can eat high fat diets and not get hardening of their arteries. Sedentary workers—from bank presidents to file clerks—just don't burn up enough energy in their daily work to be protected from the high fat diet we all habitually eat.

As physicians, we know that hardening of the arteries is related to deposits of fats within these arteries. Our sedentary living and high fat diets are too often a fatal combination.

Recently the American Medical Association Council on Foods and Nutrition came out with a program for the regulation of dietary fat. It is such a diet—which includes satisfying snacks and diet holidays—that we outline for you in this book.

YOUR APPETITE DECREASES

It is peculiar that exercise should be thought of as increasing appetite in the United States. Peculiar, because every nation in Europe regards exercise as a necessary addition to reducing appetite and improving diet, and we should regard it in this way, too.

The exercise we have talked about above is going to decrease your appetite and not increase it. The people who complain that appetite is increased by exercise are the weekend athletes who should never be listened to. Studies have shown a steady reduction in appetite occurs whenever a regular physical activity program is followed.

You will notice the same effects yourself within a few short weeks. You will eat less, not more, food when you do these exercises. But you will be more, not less, comfortable with this program. And you will realize more, not less, satisfaction from every day of your life.

Chapter Seven

EXERCISE WITHOUT MOTION—ITS BASIC PRINCIPLES

If we are to exercise correctly, we must understand what the fundamental principles of all exercises are. Once these principles are clear, each of us can evaluate the value of any specific exercise, or of any exercise program.

WHAT WE WANT FROM EXERCISE

Strength, agility and endurance are the three principle goals we wish to attain through exercise. Let us examine them, one by one.

Since no exercise can be done well without strength, much study has been devoted to strength's attainment. There have been dozens of wrong roads taken in the search for strength alone. Some of them retain their interest, since they still are accepted as truth in our own day. Here are some of the most dangerous, along with their fundamental mistakes.

During the time of the Grecian Olympics, the "training table" was invented. At such a table the wrestlers were fed a special diet, and its benefits were manifested when these specially-fed athletes won most of their contests.

The reasons for this special feeding, and its results, were quite simple. In those golden days there were no weight classifications, and in wrestling the heavier opponent always had an advantage. But once we know the reason for the training table—weight alone—it loses much of its magic.

NO WEIGHT-LIFTING

Scientific studies beginning after World War II showed that weight lifting, or progressive resistance exercises, were a superior method of gaining strength. There are dozens of books and booklets available on specific weight lifting exercises for each major sport and activity. But, like the training table, the time for their major usefulness is gone.

If weight lifting is to be done satisfactorily and safely, a trainer or coach must be available at all times to set the requirements of each day's effort. And, of course, quite a collection of gadgets are needed.

Worst of all, most weight lifters do not undertake any other exercises, but build only strength. And strength alone is only one of the three goals of exercise.

A NEW KIND OF EXERCISE

Perhaps even more effective exercises for strength have been found in *the isometric technique.*

In this form of exercise, you simply pit your own muscles against each other for a single, brief, maximum effort. Since no machinery is used, there is no possibility of overdoing.

Research has shown that this isometric technique yields two great advantages:

1) The greatest increase in strength occurs when this single maximum muscular effort is met and sustained up to no more than 6 to 10 seconds. Yes, recent research has shown that an effort of six (6) seconds per exercise is all that is needed.

2) This increase builds up the fastest when this form of exercise is used only on alternate days.

A "MILITARY" SECRET

As a matter of fact, these isometric exercises are so effective that before the recent Olympics their discovery was "blacked out"—censored as too valuable to be released—by the Western nations. Through these revolutionary new methods we hoped to crush the Russians in the Olympic game scores. No one—but no one—was going to let the Russians in on this great discovery!

Can you imagine our chagrin, when, at the beginning of the contests, all countries were found to be on an equal footing! For the Russians knew and used the same principles of isometric exercising at least as well, if not better, than did the contestants from the West. And they, of course, had kept them a "military secret" for months!

Isometric exercises are truly a revolution in quick, easy strength-building. You will discover this for yourself when you try them as described in the next chapter.

WHAT ABOUT AGILITY?

There are many kinds of exercise for agility. But agility, in itself, is not the average reader's concern; it is mainly the problem of the Olympic and professional athlete.

Agility is simply a speedy, swift muscular response—automatically correct for a particular athletic situation. This is a desirable attainment for all; but it takes a great deal of time and effort to train our bodies and minds to work together to this degree of harmony. Therefore, for the purposes of this book, we will disregard it.

HOW TO BUILD UP ENDURANCE

Endurance training—the great goal of all fitness-for-longevity programs—is accomplished by a method exactly the reverse of strength training. A great number of repetitions of minimal muscular effort are needed to gain endurance.

Purposeful walking, jogging and running stand very high on the list of good endurance training measures. They utilize the entire body. Specific techniques of walking and running will be given later.

NO PARAPHENALIA—NO CALISTHENICS

But what kind of gross omission has occurred here? There is no mention of Indian clubs, pulleys, gym suits or all of the paraphenalia we feel we must have to know that exercise is taking place.

Calisthenics are a good form of exercise, but they are time consuming, require the presence of an instructor, and require a great deal of equipment (to function satisfactorily).

Or to put it another way—they do not meet today's demands for efficiency. The time spent in going to and from the gymnasium, changing into special clothes and showering, can change a practical fitness program into a luxury that only a few can indulge in. Therefore, there are no calisthenics in this book. We substitute, instead, the far easier, simpler isometric exercises.

A NOTE OF WARNING

As a matter of fact, there are some calisthenic exercises that have no place in any fitness programs—whether that program is designed for twenty year old youths, or for those in their eighties.

Deep knee bends are foremost on the list of those exercises that are completely wrong. The knee is the most easily damaged joint in our bodies, and the hardest to heal. A half, or modified knee bend will place all the work on the leg muscles that is needed to give them either strength or endurance. More bending only adds a dangerous load on the knee joint—far more than it was built to endure. A dislocation or torn ligament may easily result.

Push-ups are for kids; so are chinning exercises. As we pass out of our twenties we invite disaster with any type of exercise that can make us hold our breath while straining. When we engage in a forceful activity—and at the same time stop regular breathing—we also stop the flow of blood into the right side of the heart. The older we are, the more this is apt to cause a heart attack.

Too many of the exercises in vogue today are aimed only at development of the extremities. Instead, by concentrating on running and walking, plus a schedule with the jump rope and isometrics, we will take sufficient care of all parts of our bodies.

We live in our torso, yet too few exercises are designed to increase the strength of its muscles. The program outlined here will give balanced activity to our trunk and our arms and legs without turning us into sideshow types.

NO UGLY BULGES

Remember, a correct posture, good muscle tone, a balanced diet and a balanced life are all we need for the essentials of life.

Incidentally, don't worry about bulging muscles from this program—they will not appear. Your muscles and other tissues will firm up and improve in appearance, but they won't bulge. For many this new firmness will bring some slight added weight, but no added fat at all.

This new, attractive appearance applies as much to women as to men. If this sounds unbelievable, simply look at any woman performer in her sixties or even eighties still traveling with a circus as an aerialist, high wire performer, or other type of gymnast. She will look more feminine and attractive than many a gal forty years her junior. And think of the money she saves by not having to purchase new foundation garments every season!

WHAT TIME OF DAY SHOULD YOU DO THESE EXERCISES?

There has been a great deal of magical thinking associated with the idea of exercising at some particular time of day. The different times of day recommended by various "experts" cover our entire waking hours—and mean nothing. It always seems best to do anything—exercise included—when you feel like it, and to avoid the same activity when you don't. A physical fitness program only needs to be done to be useful; the time of day has no more bearing on the end results than do the tides or the stars. Three half hours a week, at any time you wish. But do them.

Incidentally, experience has demonstrated that all exercises are most useful when done to rhythm. Long before the scientists could confirm this in their laboratories, men and women who did muscular work were applying this knowledge in folk songs and sailors chanteys.

You may be able to put on your phonograph when exercising, or you may only be able to give yourself the accompaniment of a 1, 2, 3, 4, count. Either rhythm will help you swing through your paces.

POINTS TO WATCH

Throughout any exercise program, of course, certain precautionary directions must be constantly kept in mind:

(1) No one should ever exercise to the point of exhaustion. Olympic athletes, who are today breaking all past records, have discovered that training short of the point of exhaustion gives them far better results than if they train to exhaustion.

They have also learned to regard the warnings of sudden exhaustion, and so rest for several days, if they have become exhausted, before resuming their training program.

(2) Other precautions that should be observed are these signs that exercising has been too strenuous:

(a) Your heart refuses to stop pounding 10 minutes after exercising.

(b) Your breathing is still uncomfortable 10 minutes after exercising.

(c) You are still shaky for more than 30 minutes after exercising.

(d) You cannot sleep well the night after exercising.

(e) You carry fatigue (not muscle soreness) into the next day.

If any of these symptoms occur, reduce the number of exercises you do by one third, and build up gradually to the former figure over a week or two.

Chapter Eight

SPECIFIC EXERCISES

In your training program the isometric exercises should be done first. Each of the following group of seven exercises requires one maximum muscle effort of six seconds or less three times a week. Only do less if your muscles cannot sustain the six second time limit. The sign of muscle fatigue is shakiness of the arms or legs during the exercise.

Now, let us start to develop the kind of body we have always dreamed about:

MUSCLE-STRENGTHENING EXERCISE NO. 1

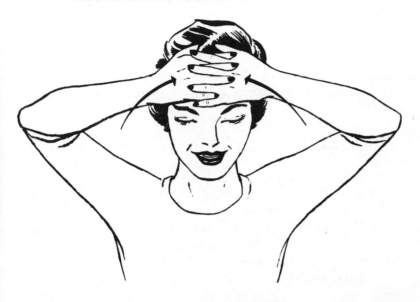

FOR THE HEAD AND NECK MUSCLES

Place your hands with interlocked fingers upon your forehead. The hands should attempt to push head back out of the way, while the head pushes forward.

MUSCLE-STRENGTHENING EXERCISE NO. 2

FOR SHOULDERS, ARMS AND NECK

1. Place the left hand against the left side of your head and push as hard as possible, trying to push the head onto your right shoulder. Resist this pressure with your neck muscles.

2. Place the right hand against the right side of your head and try to push your head onto your right shoulder. Resist with your neck muscles.

A brief rest period may be taken after each of these exercises.

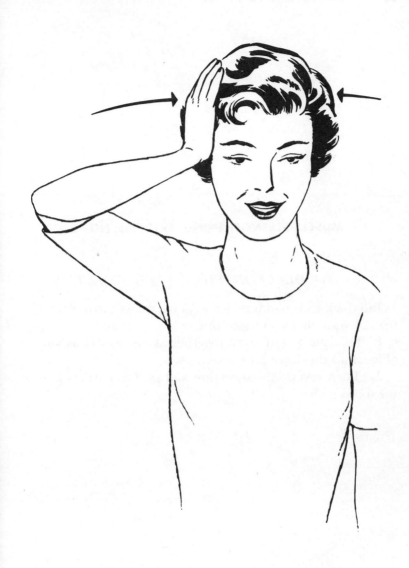

MUSCLE-STRENGTHENING EXERCISE NO. 3

TO DEVELOP THE UPPER CHEST

Interlock your hands or wrists at chest level with your arms up and your elbows straight out.

1. First push your arms together as vigorously as you are able. Hold this force for six seconds.

2. Then reverse the direction and pull as hard as possible for six seconds.

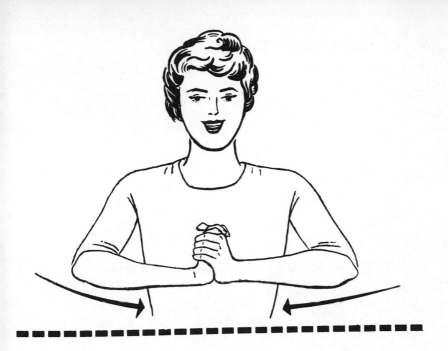

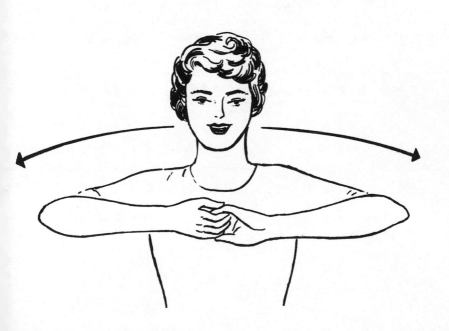

MUSCLE-STRENGTHENING EXERCISE NO. 4

TO DEVELOP ARMS, SHOULDERS, LEGS, THIGHS AND MID-SECTION

While semi-seated, hold the ends of a rope (Five to eight feet long depending on your size) firmly in each hand. At the same time, hold the loop of the rope against the soles of your feet.

Press against the rope as vigorously as possible with both feet, and attempt to pull your feet up with the rope.

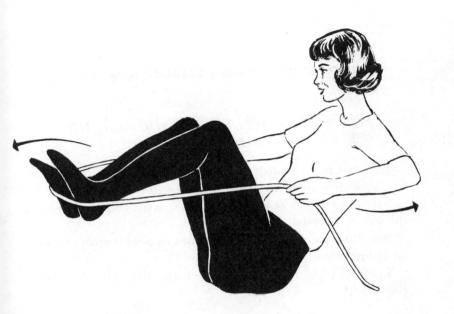

MUSCLE-STRENGTHENING EXERCISE NOS. 5 & 6

FOR THE MIDSECTION, ABDOMEN, HIPS AND THIGHS

#5. Assume a seated position on the floor before a door frame, with your feet resting in the center of the frame.

Attempt to push out the door frame with your feet, letting the structure resist.

#6. Shift your position to a corner of a wall with one foot on either side of the wall.

Squeeze your legs together, letting the structure resist your effort.

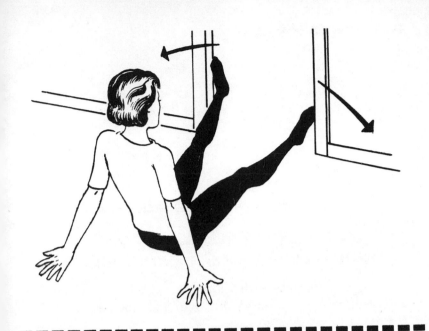

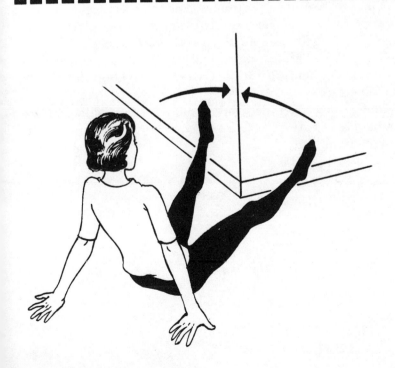

MUSCLE-STRENGTHENING EXERCISE NO. 7

TO DEVELOP THE LEGS AND SHOULDERS

Stand in a doorway with your hands against the frame and your feet well braced and the right foot forward.

Push as hard as you can.

Then reverse your position so that the left leg takes the position of the right leg, the left arm takes the place of the right. Push, again, as hard as you can for 6 seconds.

Remember: Performing each of these exercises three times a week is sufficient; five times a week is maximum for health and longevity.

Doing these exercises three times a week will increase strength at a rate of 5% a week, and then maintain it at maximum for life.

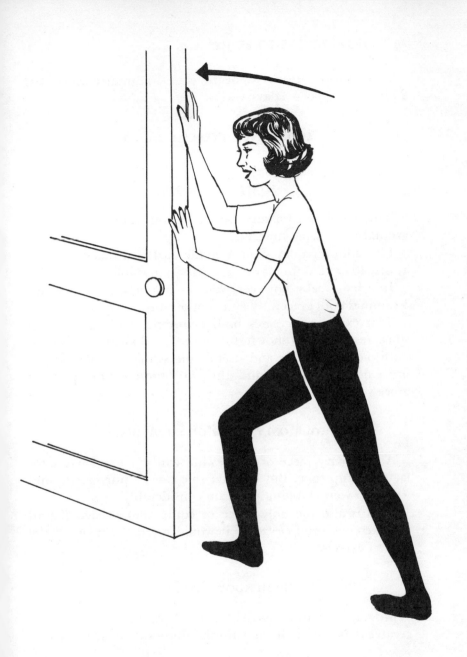

Now you are ready to begin your Endurance Exercises: 25 minutes a day—3 days a week.

ENDURANCE EXERCISE NO. 1

JUMPING ROPE

Throw the rope forward, and have both your feet leave the ground at the same time.

Five minutes a day should be the goal of this activity. But at first 10 or 12 skips may be all that are possible.

In a few weeks, however, you can anticipate jumping for 5 minutes both gracefully and comfortably.

This exercise increases both endurance and agility. And since research has shown that exercise done to rhythm is both more enjoyable and useful, the swinging rope will set up a definite rhythm and this will promote the physical grace you are striving after.

YOUR ONLY PIECE OF EQUIPMENT

An ordinary piece of clothesline will make a fairly satisfactory jump rope. But a better one can be purchased—and will help your skipping program considerably.

This is also the only piece of equipment needed for all the exercises—and certainly it would merit the name of the perfect exerciser.

TREMENDOUS BENEFITS

Most important of all, the rewards of jumping rope are greater than we might first think. Studies done at the Lank-

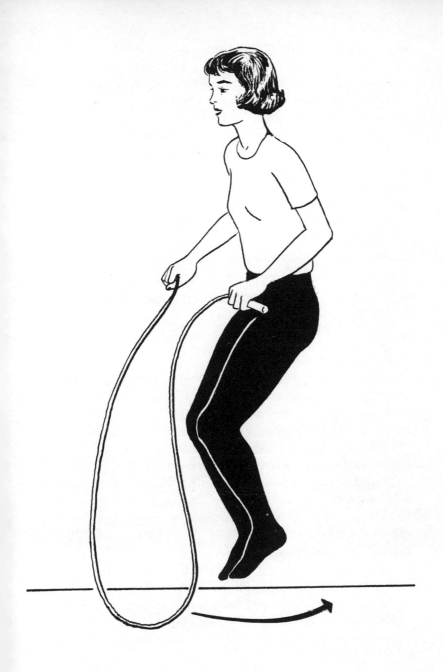

enau Hospital in Philadelphia have shown a *one hundred sixty-eight per cent increase in endurance* in six weeks training with the jump rope alone!

The group studied were normal, young, flabby Americans —you and I! When they were told of the results, and felt within themselves the benefits of this simple fitness program, they continued it without the slightest urging or reasoning from anyone.

Also, if you want to do some *daily* exercise this is the best one to do. It only takes five minutes and can be done anywhere.

ENDURANCE EXERCISE NO. 2

RUNNING

Either running or swimming 20 minutes each exercise day should be your eventual goal.

Because of weather, time and other factors, it is easier to start a running program than a swimming program. Under the worst circumstances you can run in place in your own bedroom if there is no other spot available.

Of course, few of us can carry out a full program of twenty minutes running immediately. At first you should walk briskly and vigorously for ten minutes, then fifteen minutes, then twenty minutes to loosen the muscles and build endurance for running.

Once twenty minutes of vigorous walking has been accomplished, trotting should be undertatken. Trot for two, three or four minutes and walk for an equal length of time until a twenty minute period has elapsed.

As you progress in your fitness, some of the trotting can

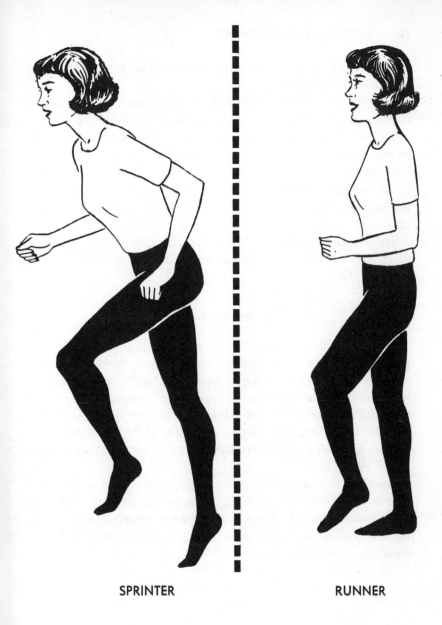

SPRINTER   RUNNER

be sped up to a good running pace with periods of walking and trotting as before.

At the end of three or four months, twenty minutes of continuous running should be possible without effort.

Always try to run in the long, easy, rather flat-footed stride of the marathon runner, rather than the snappy, ball-of-the-foot stride of the sprint runner. This sprint-runner style causes additional strain and does not in any way add to the endurance changes that occur in the body doing the easier trot.

Incidentally, other activities may be substituted for running, and we will discuss those in future chapters, especially Chapter IX.

A WORD OF CAUTION

Walking city streets with cars and stop lights slowing our pace and giving us prolonged rest periods does not build endurance. Either walking or running should be carried out in an area where this type of slow-down will not occur. The distance traveled does not have a great deal to do with the usefulness of the exercise. Exploring different routes, of course, increases enjoyment and helps us mentally as well as physically.

Another misconception people frequently have is that they can do the half-hour program over a day in little five-and-ten-minute sections. This is completely wrong. Exercise, to be useful and build strength and endurance, must be both continuous and strenuous.

Chapter Nine

YOUR NEW STYLE OF WALKING

How did you learn to walk? Did you go to a school where experts on body mechanics were in regular attendance? That would, no doubt, be the best way to learn this essential part of daily living. But I don't think that there is any such school even now, and we know that no such education was thought of at the time we learned to walk.

We learned to walk, unfortunately, by imitation. Most of those whom we imitated were too tired to care, either how they stood, or how they walked; and certainly they did not realize that they were acting as examples.

So we grew up walking with their slouch, their slumped shoulders, their protruding stomach and all their fatigue, sore feet, and aching backs.

So now we have to learn to walk all over again—the right way. It's easy; it uses far less energy; and it pays big dividends in comfort and strength for every part of our bodies.

THE FIRST STEP—STANDING CORRECTLY

Before we can walk correctly we must stand correctly. Then as we walk we will find out that by having our standing posture correct, our walking posture will be easier and more natural.

Dramatic proof of this fact will become apparent the day after you have started this new method of locomotion. Out of the habit of years you will begin to stand and walk the old way. But then in a few minutes you will realize that you are working too hard, and you will shift into the new position as a matter of comfort.

Then, without doing anything else, you will be surprised to find your friends telling you how well you look, and even asking you how you "lost weight." Even if you haven't lost an ounce, it is nice to know you are carrying your weight better.

HERE WE GO, THEN—

It is easy to learn to stand the right way. Here's all you do:

Stand up against a wall—we have all heard this—then simply flatten the small of your back against that wall.

What happens? Your pelvis goes toward the wall at the top, and comes out, away from the wall at the bottom. Your tail is tucked away toward the back of your legs and your tummy goes in. You feel thinner immediately, and you show it.

To do this muscle movement correctly, you must keep your knees locked and your heels touching the wall throughout the exercise.

After you have achieved the proper stance, tighten up all

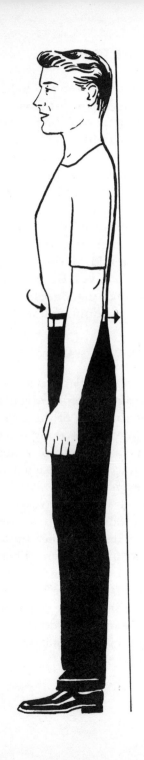

the muscles that you are using to hold it. Five or ten colored pictures would not show you the right muscles to tighten in this position. But your own body will tell you when you've got them lined up right. Now hold them for six seconds, and relax.

This posture exercise can be done in the same fashion, at the same time, as the other isometric exercises; if you need strength for correct posture, as most of us do, it will perform wonders in a few short weeks.

Like any other isometric exercise, this maximum tensing of these muscles should be done no more often than every other day, and three days a week is sufficient for a good gain in strength. Not that the muscles should be flabby in between—just not at maximum effort.

A PERSON WHO WALKS WELL, LOOKS WELL

"Lift up your feet, Soldier!" is a command that many men have had beat against their eardrums, but few have heard. Yet this is an essential part of the correct method of walking.

Most of us push one foot along the ground, while we slide the other foot into a position for a new push. That's neither the easy nor the graceful way to get around.

Our posture exercise, while standing at the wall, is the beginning of good walking. Now, to take your first step towards this new walk, don't push away from that wall. Instead, *lift up* your leg from the thigh. Move it upward and forward, and then put it down. Then *lift up* the other leg from the thigh, and put it down. *This* is good walking.

It may help to *lift* up your leg if you concentrate on the muscles in the front of your leg from your pelvis to your knee. These are the ones that do the lifting.

Now, walk around the room two or three times this new

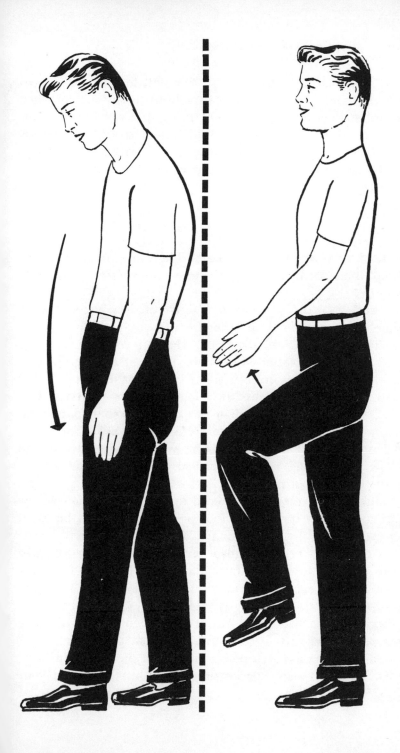

way and come back to the wall. You will find that a surprising thing has happened; your back is much flatter than when you first stood at that wall. Or, to say it another way, your posture—both standing and walking—is straighter. To get the most grace and comfort in your new walking you should make sure that your knees nearly touch as they pass each other.

TIPS ON FOOT COMFORT

Look at your toes as you walk. The more nearly you can keep them pointed straight ahead, the better your walk will be.

Check your shoes. An even slightly run-down heel on your shoe can keep you from straightening out your foot to the desired straight-ahead direction. Have it replaced at once.

A pair of moccasins—not shoes, but real moccasins—will help you learn the correct style of walking. Put them on and walk around on the grass for a few moments—and you will quickly learn why the Indian was known as sure footed and quiet of step. In these comfortable foot protectors your balance depends on coordinating your muscles as you go along. A shuffling step is punished by losing either a moccasin, or your footing.

Moccasins give another reward to our feet: we can wiggle our toes. Many of us have foot problems that can be eased or even helped by using our toes more in walking.

A commonly recommended exercise for weak or sore feet is to pick up your socks from the floor with your bare feet several times each day. Many with foot problems find that they can't do this seemingly simple task even once! A little practice, and a little time out of hard-soled shoes will make the toes sufficiently flexible to accomplish this trick.

Another method is to pick a marble off the floor with your toes. This will also exercise the muscles in the rest of your feet.

Too many of us walk all day long with our toes in an almost paralysed position. The more flexibility we develop in our feet the more comfort we will have in walking—and even running will become enjoyable instead of being a task.

YOU REAP DIVIDENDS EVERY DAY OF YOUR LIFE

There is even a slight economic advantage to this style of walking: the heels on your shoes won't wear out nearly so fast! Since you are lifting, not pushing your foot, it comes down flat on the ground. Very little weight is placed on your heel. The ball of your foot will begin to come alive, and your toes will feel more active than they have been for years.

The rest of your posture will automatically take care of itself. Chin in, chest out, etc. Much more important, you will want to start that program of regular daily walking that you know you must begin.

Now is the time to make that commitment. Commit, not just promise. Commit yourself to a healthy life with the knowledge that it will be a long and happy one.

Chapter Ten

OPTIONAL EXERCISES—FOR THOSE WHO WISH TO DO MORE THAN THE MINIMUM PROGRAM

In the last two chapters we went over a basic maintenance program of exercises. This minimum program will get you in shape and keep you there. But many readers will want to know what further exercises they can do during the day to wake themselves up—to put even more vigor into their future.

THE EUROPEAN EXERCISE BREAK

As I have said, in Sweden the coffee break has been replaced by the exercise break. Some examples of these stand-up, quick, easy-to-do exercises are given below.

Another country, Russia, has also adopted these rest-break exercises with a strong affirmative. Manpower, particularly skilled manpower, is not to be thrown away lightly in the economy of the U. S. S. R. Exercise, to the Russians, is as much a weapon of national policy as rockets.

1) "QUIET EXERCISES"

Yet, in our country, exercise is looked upon with greater disdain than is alcoholism—Why? Because of the supposed necessity of lying on a floor, devoting hours to each exercise period, changing into new clothes, etc.

Quiet exercises are the answer that most of us need if we want to do more than the minimum program without fuss or bother. These can be done while attending a meeting, operating a lathe, or going over to the watercooler.

With this method of exercise, we simply make our muscles tense for a brief moment and relax them.

For example, you can make the muscles of your left leg tight for a moment, then let these muscles go limp as you tense the muscles of your right leg. This can be done while you are standing or sitting. But don't try to do it while walking, as you may either throw yourself off stride, or cause a muscle cramp.

Tightening and relaxing the muscles of your arms and of your abdomen can be done at almost any time, and no one will ever be aware of your activity.

If you add muscle tightening activities to your back muscles, however, you certainly will be noticed, since this activity will force you into a better posture.

The most dramatic example I ever had of the value of these quiet exercises occurred one afternoon when several of us were in a meeting with the long-time Commissioner of Health in Chicago, the late Dr. Herman Bundesen. After about a half hour he leaped up from behind his desk and told us that while we had all been sitting and growing more flabby he had spent the same time in quiet exercise.

At that time he was seventy-five, worked from eight in the

morning until about six at night, attended numerous night meetings—and still dared us all to a stair climbing race. His challenge was not accepted—not because of respect for his age but because of our own certainty of loss.

Quiet exercises, walking and running were the major physical activities that Dr. Bundesen used to maintain excellent health during his lifetime. They can be an equally powerful weapon in your own armory of fitness.

2) YOUR OWN "EXERCISE-BREAK"

Exercise should not only be made respectable, but part of our daily life. All of us know the social and health necessity of brushing our teeth and bathing, yet few of us think of exercise in the same way. We should learn to think of fitness as being at least as much a part of our daily grooming as are the other parts of our health rituals.

Why not adapt the Swedish exercise break to your own office routine? Why not substitute such an exercise break for the gossip and coffee session that most of us have in our work? A phonograph is simply set up, the leader assumes his place, and mild, dignified exercises begin right at the desks.

The exercises are all comfortable and require no special equipment or costumes for full participation. For many reasons, there are no push-ups, pull-ups, knee-bends or other outmoded styles of mock heroic activities. All of these movements are done in the standing position, and principally involve the trunk and arms.

FUN AND HEALTH AT THE OFFICE

A description of eight of these work-break activities is included here so that you, Mr. Plant and Mrs. Office Director, can start your own group on this extra-health program. Morale, vitality and efficiency, as well as longevity, will be the rewards of your staffs.

Exercise 1—Stand up. Place your hands on your hips and rotate your head, shoulders and upper trunk as a unit in a slight circle. Do this eight times.

Exercise 2—Swing your right hand and arm in an up-and-down circle at the side of the body. Do this five times. Then do the same exercise with your left arm.

Exercise 3—With your arms again on your waist, alternately kick out to 15 degrees or 20 degrees, first with your left, then with your right leg. Do this ten to twenty times.

Exercise 4—While standing, bring the hands in front of the body and bend down to touch some part of the leg between the knees and the ankles. Do this five times. No attempt should be made to touch the floor with the finger tips as this often puts too much strain on the back.

Exercise 5—While standing with the arms straight at the sides, rotate the head in a circle trying to touch the shoulders with the ears. Make a full circle five times.

Exercise 6—Place the hands at the side and roll the shoulders about their center five times.

Exercise 7—While standing, place the hands in front with the fingers gripping imaginary oars. Bring the hands diagonally up to the shoulders in a rowing motion. This can be done five to ten times.

Exercise 8—Stand on your toes and reach for the ceiling with your arms. Pause a moment, then come back down on your feet. Do this five times.

All these exercises can be done in ordinary clothes and in conventional postures; no special equipment is needed, nor is a great deal of extra space necessary.

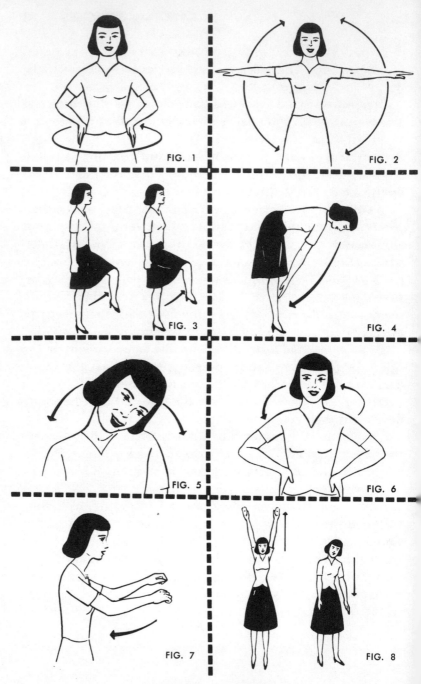

WORK-BREAK EXERCISES

3) BREATHING EXERCISES

Breathing exercises have been in and out of vogue since the early 1800's. They can serve as an excellent non-caloric form of refreshment as well as giving our muscles some much needed motion. Here are two of the best:

Exercise 1—Sit in a chair with the feet about nine inches apart. Lean forward and hold the front legs of the chair. In this position inhale and exhale deeply. Repeat three or four times and rest. Since this position fixes the muscles of the shoulders, all the breathing effort will be done by the abdominal musculature.

Exercise 2—Lean back in an armchair and press the shoulders against it. Stretch the feet out in front on a hassock. Again, take three or four deep breaths for this exercise, and rest.

OTHER FORMS OF EXERCISE-RECREATION

All the exercises in this chapter are designed to be done by anyone who does not have some severe physical handicap. By adding these to the maintenance program of exercise, you can continue to improve your muscular tone and your mental outlook.

Not only are all these optional exercises helpful, but there are many good modern-dancing classes for adults which also result in a great deal of exercise. In this day of suburban living and civic activities there are many such opportunities open to nearly all of us.

Although not every swimming pool in the country is open twelve months of the year, there are certainly a great number of pools available everywhere. Swimming vigorously and continuously for twenty minutes can do just as much for our physical fitness as running for an equal amount of time.

In each area of the country there are unique sporting opportunities. These should be used for variety and pleasure in your fitness program. We shall discuss them in the next chapter.

Chapter Eleven

RECREATION AND SPORTS

The exercise program outlined in the previous chapters is a minimum fitness schedule that we all should follow. Most of us can do more. Sports bring us out of doors and give us a variety of physical activity that prevents boredom. They also give our minds new challenges with attendant pleasure at their solution.

After a period of difficult work the change to satisfying sports can do far more to refresh us than any number of hours of sleep, or of passing time watching the activities of others in a ball park or on a TV screen. Let's look at some of the best of them:

CAMPING

Camping and hiking are still far less used for recreation than they should be. Physically they give us many opportunities for refreshing activities. Mentally they give us an even greater change in outlook, often with new companions and experiences that we could never find in our routine living.

Exposure to the elements is also beneficial to both body and soul. Nor are these sights and pleasures the sole property of the very rich of the world. Short trips by bus or car will bring anyone to a spot in the country where nature can be both enjoyed and studied.

Outdoor living, including moderate exposures to wind, sun, cold, water, and natural hours of sleep following hard work, should be followed for at least two weeks every year. At least one vacation a year should be devoted to camping, supplemented by weekends of hiking, swimming, archery or shooting, sailing, boating, canoeing, fishing, nature study, skiing or climbing.

HIKING

Certainly the easiest way to get out of doors is to go hiking. You can participate in this wonderfully beneficial sport in your own neighborhood—or, if you wish, travel thousands of miles to some particularly beautiful area.

LITTLE EQUIPMENT IS NEEDED

The equipment needed for hiking can be bought for a surprisingly low price, and will return its cost many times over in the comfort it brings.

A good pair of shoes certainly is first on the list. For a man, a pair of work oxfords can be purchased at a reasonable price that will give a great deal of wear. Since these shoes should be worn with a pair of heavy socks, they should be fitted over the socks. A composition sole with a pattern is best to give good footing when in the woods. High shoes and boots are not comfortable to wear on most hiking tours, as they bend and chafe the leg and cut off ventilation.

A woman's shoe and sock problem is not greatly different from a man's. She can have a choice of a low or medium heel in the same style of composition sole recommended above.

The rest of the clothing should be a combination of personal taste, personal budget, and geography.

A lightweight cotton windbreaker, sufficiently inconspicuous on warm days, can also give real protection from sudden rains and chilling winds.

A woolen shirt of appropriate weight is probably the most all-around useful item that any hiker can have for any but the hottest days. A good wool will have a surprising degree of water resistance and warmth.

Loose trousers for men, slacks for women, are the most useful leg garments. Not jeans or riding togs. Any tightly-fitted garment will bind and turn a hike into an endurance contest.

This is all the clothing anyone needs for an enjoyable hike—provided you bring along sufficient fitness for the walk itself.

FOOD, WATER, SHELTER

Nobody wants to go hiking before breakfast—so there is no need to worry about the preparation of this meal for a hike. Everything you will need for one hearty meal in the woods can be carried in a small shoulder strap bag which can be anything from a one dollar surplus gas-mask canvas bag, to a fancy leather and wicker hamper fancily priced. The food will taste the same from both.

A canteen or plastic bottle for water is always handy to have on a hike—even if no cooking is planned. Thirst is an unpleasant sensation that can grow into quite a problem when no relief is available.

In fact, about three years ago, with much planning and the

help of every conceivable expert, one of our stratospheric balloonists almost proved with his life that a little water is a valuable asset. During the night prior to the ascent, this man, busy with preparations for the ascent, did not drink any liquids. As the flight began, he became thirsty. But no water had been provided and he completed the flight with far more courage than comfort.

At the time of his descent, his fever was so high that there was real alarm for his life. He barely survived, so all balloonists now take a goodly drink of water before they launch, and include a supply of water for their trips.

The hiker's problems are far less than the spaceman's; but to most of us they can seem equally bad when we want the simplest of life's requirements—and find they are not there to be had.

NO NEED TO "ROUGH IT"

A compass is another item that anyone who walks off the streets into the smallest wood should have and know how to use. It takes up no real space, costs little, and can save your life.

A neat gadget is a plastic tube that contains a compass, a whistle, and waterproof matches. Slide one of these into your bag or pocket and you will get home.

Also tuck in a book on the woods, its trees, birds, or plants. Every hike should be punctuated by rest—and our minds can be made happier by learning more about the beauty around us than by stewing about last week's problems at work.

All this talk about equipment doesn't add up to "roughing it," and it's not supposed to. Only a green-horn, a tenderfoot, or a similar misguided person tries to rough it out. Hiking with a modicum of gear is fun; walking about with no preparation is a temptation the fates might not be able to resist.

HOW TO COOK LUNCH

Dehydrated soups and instant tea and coffee are easy to carry and give us the warmth we all want with any meal. Heating the water can be done in many ways.

A wood fire from sticks is more a dream than a reality. Most of it is so wet you need a blowtorch to dry it out. Canned heat provides a better way to warm a little food and water quickly.

Pocket stoves by the dozen are for sale and nearly all of them do the job they are supposed to. If you want the fuels most of them need, you must know their special names and the places to get them. Kerosene may be purchased in a gas station by asking for diesel fuel. White gas is obtained at the hardware store by ordering naphtha. And alcohol, very strangely, is sold under its own name!

Food of the very best flavor and variety is available in nearly any sporting goods store. Frozen, dry, dehydrated foods are available in such variety as almost to cause confusion. The grocery man also has many of these foods, in addition to his regular lines of appetite satisfiers.

Always make sure that you read the instructions on the box before you are out in the woods, or disappointments are sure to occur. "Season to taste"—not if the salt and pepper are back home. "Add one egg"—who carries eggs on a hike? Or "Put in one-half cup of milk." The price of being unprepared comes rather high in flat, thin, tasteless food when the pantry is far away.

All in all, a sandwich and soup can be quite enough for many hikers. For those that want to spend a little more time in preparation, a full meal is easy to prepare. Bring along a small pan or two, paper plates and napkins, and you'll be able to put your knife and fork to good use.

TRUE HEALTH—TRUE DEMOCRACY

To repeat, camping, the next step up from hiking, is an inexpensive method of sightseeing, and a nice way to become acquainted with many fine people that you would not meet in any other way. In camping we can come closest to the French conception of a democracy, for Liberty, Fraternity, and Equality are all found in camping.

It is harder to advise a person on the proper camping equipment to use than to advise him on a marriage partner, because tastes are so individual. In the case of camping equipment, a happy solution can be found in the many fine stores that rent such equipment. By trial, some errors, and good council from these stores, it is possible to find out what you like in camp gear and buy it to suit your convenience. Since there are several good books on camping, I will not repeat their advice here.

OTHER SPORTS

Although most of us can go for some sort of hike in the woods, less of us are able to take off for swimming, sailing, skiing and other elite sports. Those who are able to afford these recreational opportunities—and fortunately this includes more of us every year—should not pass them by, but should use them as a means of increasing their fitness and their enjoyment of life.

However, some sports are deliberately left out in this chapter—for definite reasons.

Many no longer contribute to fitness or health. Golf, played only in fine weather, with the cart to save every useful step, is fine recreation, but not a sport. Bowling—where an entire night is spent getting through two lines—is equally impoverished as a sport.

Some sports are omitted because not everyone is in good enough shape to indulge in them with safety. Handball can be dangerous when the competition gets too keen and the players ignore the warning signs of exhaustion. I have seen enough heart attacks in thirty to forty year old players to make me want to caution against too hard a game.

Tennis and squash are also only for the fit—not for those wildly hoping to prove their stories of the glories of yester-year.

Body contact sports are not needed in any fitness program, and I leave their discussion for the professional athletes and their trainers and coaches.

RECREATION AND FITNESS

Not all recreation must contribute to fitness, of course, but why shouldn't we get as much fitness out of our recreation as humanly possible?

Playing a different sport each season will add to fun and companionship. Our bodies will gain a new vitality through exposure to the weather—a glow and vigor they can never acquire in the protection of controlled warmth during winter and air conditioning in summer.

"Take it easy" is only good advice if you have been doing something hard. Most of us sit all day, then rush home to lie down in preparation for going to bed. That schedule is not easy, it's deadly. Deadly in terms of boredom, and in terms of death itself, long before death should be our lot.

TUNE UP YOUR BODY

We all know that our cars must be tuned up at regular intervals. And most of them need to be given a fairly good high speed run at times, to keep from getting all stuck up with carbon and gum. Yet the idea of a good high speed walk, even a moderately uncomfortable one, seems out of the question for most of us.

These research findings, presented in the publication *Physical Fitness for Adults* by the President's Council on Youth Fitness, should be taken to heart by all who are interested in a healthy life:

"that (1) A sound heart cannot be damaged by exercise; (2) that more heart and circulatory troubles result from too mild and too short exercise periods; and (3) that exercise is needed to normalize the blood chemistry in the face of higher fat consumption in modern diets."

Don't build a wall of civilized comforts about yourself. Get out into the weather occasionally and live—longer and better.

Chapter Twelve

A NEW DIET FOR YOUR NEW LIFE

In a recent issue of the *Journal of the American Medical Association* there is a report from the Council on Foods and Nutrition called "Regulation of Dietary Fat." (Now published by the A.M.A. as a booklet with this title.)

The many authors of this study state that this is a guide to the physician who wishes to advise and regulate dietary fat on the basis that it may be beneficial. "It is not a recommendation for the general public." However, this highly accurate and technical article should be of interest to all of us who wish to live a long life and avoid disease.

MEET THE KILLERS

This report confirms what we have already stated in this book. 25% to 30% of all deaths in the United States are due to heart attacks alone. Another 30% to 40% of United States deaths are due to other forms of hardening of the arteries. And as the American Medical Association article states, "many studies of diets in relation to mortality . . . have shown that populations that have a high rate of coronary artery disease also have high mean cholesterol values . . . subsist on diets rich in animal protein, fats and calories." This is a perfect description of the American diet today.

Another cause of death is obesity. One half the men in the United States over 35 are more than 10% overweight. *And you are ten times more likely to get a coronary if you combine this obesity with high blood fat and high blood pressure.*

HOW OVERWEIGHT SHORTENS YOUR LIFE

The table shown here presents this terrifying fact in a more graphic form. To repeat a tragic fact once more, today about one half of all males over 35 are at least 10% overweight. They do not realize that for every pound of overweight, they have decreased their life expectancy exactly 1%.

THESE KILLERS CAN BE CONTROLLED

This obesity and high blood fat can be readily controlled by using the American Medical Association's "Modified Fatty Acid Content" diet. This diet shows how much to eat to obtain 1200, 1800 and 2400 calories each day.

1200 calories would mean a stringent reduction program for nearly anyone. If you want to lose weight fast, try this diet for a week or two.

1800 calories would be a full maintenance diet for small, sedentary people and a weight reduction diet for those who are large and active. A woman doing sedentary work would probably need only 1800 calories for her daily intake. A large muscular man doing physical work might need better than twice as much to maintain his weight. If the 1200 calorie diet

WEIGHT Chart

Height In Inches	Weight You Should Be	Danger Weight	Cuts 25% Off Your Life Expectancy	Cuts 50% Off Your Life Expectancy	Cuts 75% Off Your Life Expectancy	Adds this % to his chances of dying Cuts 100% Off Your Life Expectancy
5—0	117	159	175	185	195	205
5—1	120	163	180	190	200	210
2	123	168	185	195	205	215
3	127	172	190	200	210	220
4	131	177	195	205	215	225
5	134	182	200	210	220	230
6	138	186	205	215	225	235
7	141	191	210	220	230	240
8	145	196	215	225	235	245
9	149	200	220	230	240	250
10	153	205	225	235	245	255
11	157	210	230	240	250	260
6—0	161	215	235	245	255	265
6—1	165	220	240	250	260	270
2	169	225	245	255	265	275
3	174	230	250	260	270	End
4	179	235	255	265	275	End
5	184	240	260	270	End	
6	188	245	265	275	End	
7	193	250	270	End		
8	198	255	275	End		

If your weight is over 275 you can see by the chart you have been left out! This is not an accident. Insurance companies have found out that people over this weight have dealt terrible damage to their life expectancy through their obesity.

is too stringent for you, try the 1800 calorie diet for a week or two—it may easily do the trick.

The same general thinking applies to the 2400 calorie diet. This could be a maintenance level for a fifty year old man doing sedentary work, or a weight reduction program for a lumberjack. This should be your maintenance diet once you have attained normal weight by using either the 1200 or 1800 calorie diets.

The physical fitness program outlined in this book will also help us obtain and maintain normal weight. It will not increase our appetite, and, as we mentioned before, it may even help those who have high blood pressure.

Getting to a normal weight is also frequently helpful for high blood pressure. We intend to do this by the slow and gentle weight reduction program outlined below, which will give truly thrilling results for most of us without straining any of the body's mechanisms.

These diets will also re-train the appetite and start us on new, healthier and equally comfortable dietary habits.

BASIC RULES

To obtain a reduction in calories and fat, the following principles must be achieved:

All fats, milk and nuts are excluded. Baked goods are restricted, and the use of fruits and low-fat vegetables is emphasized.

In order to increase the polyunsaturated fat in the diet, the saturated fat content must be reduced as follows:

The principal reduction of this saturated fat must come from a reduction in the two main food groups that contribute most of the saturated fat—dairy products and meats.

In all the diets the milk is nonfat, no cream is allowed

and eggs are limited to 4 per week. Only lean meats, fish and poultry are used. Chocolate and caramel-type candies made with cocoa butter should be avoided. Commercial bakery goods other than bread are excluded except for the "Diet Holidays" mentioned below.

Certain "special" table margarines should be used instead of butter or vegetable oils. There are also "special" shortenings available which have a polyunsaturated fatty acid content similar to the "special" margarines and which may be used in baked goods.

You can use any of these diets for a week or a month to trim off weight—but the 2,400 calorie diet, or some form of it, is best used for a lifetime.

Combined with regular health audit examinations, and the rules of mental and physical hygiene listed in this book, such a diet will give you a greatly increased life expectancy. And more vitality every step of the way.

Chapter Thirteen

DIETS, DIET SNACKS AND DIET HOLIDAYS

Here are some practical menus for you to follow in learning this new dietary pattern. I suggest you try one week at 1200 calories, two weeks at 1800 calories, and a fourth week at 2400 calories. Then check your weight.

Of course, this is not the ideal diet for everyone—such a diet hasn't been invented as yet. If in doubt, consult your physician first; then begin this or whatever other diet he recommends.

BUILD IN VARIETY

Incidentally, you might look over the current crop of cookbooks, and find one that will give you some new recipes to bring variety and spice to these extremely flexible diets. Remember, there are many different kinds of foods, and delightful new ways of preparing them, that will help you to stay within your calorie limits, and yet give you the freshness and variety we all crave.

EVERYONE JOINS IN

Do not try to follow these diets while everyone else at the table stuffs down the same old fat foods they have been eating for years. Everybody in the family must get into the act! When father or mother start to change their ways, that is the time for the rest of the family to go along.

WHAT ABOUT RESTAURANTS?

These diets are equally easy to follow if you eat in restaurants, if you only have a little ingenuity. These restaurants have the foods you want—for the combined reasons that they wish to please you, and stay in business. Of course there are places that seem only to serve hamburgers, but if you will take a second look at their menu, you'll find that most of them have a great deal more variety to offer. Just look and ask.

YOUR DIET HOLIDAYS

There are only six days in a dieter's week; on the seventh —like Jehovah—we should rest. It doesn't have to be any particular day of the week, but do go off the diet one day out of seven. Do it when there is a party, when something goes wrong, when you are bored, or sometimes upon no occasion at all. This one day of self-indulgence will refresh your spirit, strengthen your good humor, reward your accomplishments, and maybe even help your metabolism.

Modified Fatty Acid Diet   1200 Calories

DAY ONE

Breakfast

Grapefruit	one-half
Cereal	cooked oatmeal one-half cup
Skim milk	one cup (8 ounces)
Sweeten with sugar substitute	

Lunch

Sandwich of:

Chicken	two (2) ounces
Bread	2 slices
Special mayonnaise	1 teaspoon

Salad of:

Lettuce, celery, green pepper

Salad Dressing	teaspoon of oil with salt, pepper and vinegar to taste.
Baked Apple	small—sweeten with sugar substitute
Coffee or tea	no milk or sugar

Dinner

Haddock	3 oz. (fried in 2 teaspoons oil)
Bread	1 slice (may be used to bread haddock)
Mayonnaise	2 teaspoons (may be mixed with relish as tartar sauce)
Spinach	one-half cup
Carrots	one-half cup
Skim milk	one cup (8 ounces)
Pear	one small (cooked, canned or fresh)
Sugar	use sugar substitute

Snack

Coffee, tea or non-caloric soft
  drink

DAY TWO

Breakfast

Orange juice	Small (4 ounce) glass
Cereal	¾ cup of dry or prepared
Skim milk	one cup (8 ounces)
Sweeten with sugar substitute	
Coffee or tea	

Lunch

Sandwich of:	
Veal	two ounces
Bread	two slices
Special mayonnaise	one teaspoon
Salad of:	
Lettuce, tomatoes, radishes	
Salad dressing	one teaspoon of oil, salt, pepper, vinegar to taste
Peach	one medium (canned, fresh or cooked)
Coffee or tea	sugar substitute

Dinner

Salmon	3 ounces (broiled with 2 tea-spoons oil)
Dinner roll	one 2-inch in diameter
Special margarine	2 pats
Beans, string	one-half cup
Beets	one-half cup
Skim milk	one cup (8 ounces)
Pineapple	one-half cup (fresh or canned)
Sugar	use sugar substitute

Snack

Coffee, tea or non-caloric soft drink	

DAY THREE

Breakfast

Orange	one small
Shredded wheat biscuit	one
Skim milk	one cup (8 ounces)
Sweeten with a sugar substitute	

Lunch

Sandwich of:

Turkey	two ounces
Bread	two slices
Special mayonnaise	one teaspoon

Salad of:

Asparagus with cucumber
slices

Salad dressing	1 teaspoon of oil, salt, pepper, vinegar to taste
Applesauce	one-half cup

Dinner

Beef, lean	3 ounces
Hard roll	one 2-inch in diameter
Mushrooms	one-half cup
Onions	one-half cup
Skim milk	one cup
Cherries	10 large (fresh, cooked or canned)
Sugar	use sugar substitute

Snack

Coffee, tea or non-caloric soft
drink

DAY FOUR

Breakfast

Grape Juice	one-half cup Small (4 oz.) glass
Cereal	cooked (Cream of Wheat) one-half cup
Skim milk	one cup (8 ounces)
Sweeten with sugar substitute	

Lunch

Sandwich of:	
Chicken	2 ounces
Bread	2 slices
Special mayonnaise	one teaspoon
Salad of:	
Lettuce hearts	
Salad dressing	one teaspoon oil with salt, pepper, vinegar to taste
Strawberries	one cup with sugar substitute
Coffee or tea	no milk or sugar

Dinner

Lamb, leg	3 ounces (one medium slice)
Sauerkraut	one cup
Peas, green	one-half cup
Bread	one slice
Special margarine	2 pats
Skim milk	one cup (8 ounces)
Figs	2 large (fresh or dried)
Sugar	use sugar substitute

Snack

Coffee, tea or non-caloric beverage	

DAY FIVE

Breakfast

Orange Juice	Small (4 ounce) glass
Cereal	Dry, prepared, ¾ cup
Skim milk	one cup (8 ounces)
Sweeten with sugar substitute	

Lunch

Sandwich of:
Egg salad — 2 eggs
Bread — 2 slices
Mayonnaise — one teaspoon; mustard and other spices to taste

Salad of:
Mixed greens
Salad dressing — one teaspoon oil with salt, pepper, vinegar to taste

Banana — one-half small

Dinner

Crabmeat cakes — 3 ounces (with 2 teaspoons oil, if wanted)

Bread — one slice, use with crabmeat to make cakes

Squash, summer — one cup
Beets — one-half cup
Blueberries — two-thirds cup (fresh, frozen or canned)

Skim milk — one cup
Use sugar substitutes

Snack

Coffee, tea, or non-caloric soft drink

DAY SIX

Breakfast

Banana	one-half, small
Cereal	dry, prepared, ¾ cup
Skim milk	one cup
Sugar	use sugar substitutes

Lunch

Spaghetti	one cup
Meatless sauce	one-fourth cup
Salad:	
Watercress, escarole and green peppers	
Salad dressing	one teaspoon oil, salt, pepper, vinegar to taste

Dinner

Ham, lean trimmed	three ounces [or corned beef]
Hard roll	one 2-inch in diameter
Broccoli	one cup
Carrots	one-half cup
Skim milk	one cup
Apple	medium 2-inch diameter

Snack

Coffee, tea or non-caloric soft
  drink

THE SEVENTH DAY'S REST

Now that we have behaved ourselves at the table for six days, and seen the scales move slightly backward, we want to rejoice. Fine! This is the time to relax from the diet—but still not the time for a Bacchanalian feast!

There are a few words of caution that you must read before you express your joy through your digestive system. For the past week your body has gone along on far less food than it was used to handling. Therefore, any sudden overload at this point is going to place more strain on it than would ordinarily be the case.

A big, heavy, fat-filled meal is bound to have a number of unfortunate effects on your internal machinery. It will over-load your circulation and make your heart work harder. It will make your blood form clots more readily. It can actually cause a heart attack!

This is not theory—but confirmed fact. Every practicing physician has seen this happen to a great number of men and women having their first, second or third coronary. Let's not join that club, in which membership is so dangerous.

On the other hand, don't feel that you must celebrate your bravery in following out the diet by fasting through the seventh day. Simply do this:

Eat what you want, but not too darned much of it. Have a glass of wine with your meal—or take a highball before it. Wind up the meal with a rich pastry, if that is what you crave. But have a very, very small serving.

Depending upon how you feel, you may either repeat the 1200 calorie diet the next week, or increase it to 1800 calories. The next two weeks' diets are planned on the basis of 1800 calories—but you can make them more or less than that by using the exchange pages at the end of this chapter.

Modified Fatty Acid Diet Values   1800 Calories

DAY EIGHT

Breakfast

Grapefruit	one-half with 1 tsp. sugar
Cereal	cooked (oatmeal) with 2 tspns sugar
Skim milk	one cup
Bread (toast)	1 slice
Special margarine	1 teaspoon

Lunch

Sandwich of:	
Chicken	3 ounces
Bread	2 slices
Special mayonnaise	1 teaspoon
Salad of:	
Lettuce, tomatoes, green pepper	
Salad dressing	2 teaspoons oil with salt, pepper, vinegar to taste
Baked Apple	small with one teaspoon sugar

Dinner

Fillet of Sole	3 ounces (fried in 2 teaspoons oil)
Bread	1 slice, may be used to bread Sole
Spinach and Mushrooms	one-half cup
Carrots	one-half cup with 1 teaspoon brown sugar
Potato	one small (mashed, with one teaspoon oil)

Mayonnaise	2 teaspoons with relish to taste for tartar sauce
Skim milk	one cup
Pear	1 small (cooked, canned or fresh)
Sugar	2 teaspoons or substitute one ounce alcoholic drink

Snack

Soda crackers	3
Banana	1 small

DAY NINE

Breakfast

Orange Juice	small (four ounce) glass
Shredded wheat biscuit	one, with 2 teaspoons sugar
Skim milk	one cup
Bread (toast)	1 slice
Special margarine	one teaspoon

Lunch

Sandwich of:	
Smoked salmon	3 ounces
Rye bread	2 slices
Cream cheese	one teaspoon
Onion if wanted	
Salad of:	
Mixed greens	
Dressing	one teaspoon oil with salt, pepper, and vinegar to taste
Pineapple	one-half cup with one teaspoon of sugar

Dinner

Veal	3 ounces
Hard roll	one 2-inch diameter
Special margarine	3 teaspoons
Broccoli	one-half cup
Beets	one-half cup
Potato	one small (mashed with 1 tsp oil)
Apricots	2 medium (fresh, cooked or canned)
Skim milk	one cup
Sugar	3 teaspoons, or 1½ shot of whiskey, or 2 glasses dry wine

Snack

Graham crackers	2
Plums	2 medium (fresh, cooked or canned)

DAY TEN

Breakfast

Peach	one medium (fresh, cooked or canned)
Cereal	dry, prepared, ¾ cup with 2 tsp sugar
Skim milk	one cup
Bread (toast)	one slice
Special margarine	1 teaspoon

Lunch

Rice	one cup
Crabmeat flakes	3 ounces
Sauce	2 tsp. of oil, Curry powder or spices to taste
Salad of:	
Hearts of lettuce	
Salad dressing	one tsp. oil, salt, pepper, vinegar to taste
Tangerine	1 large (fresh, or canned)

Dinner

Beef tenderloin	3 ounces
Dinner roll	1 2-inch in diameter
Special margarine	3 tsp
Carrots	one-half cup (with 1 tsp brown sugar)
Beans, string	one-half cup
Skim milk	one cup
Strawberries	one cup (fresh, frozen or canned)
Sugar	2 tsp. or 2 glasses dry wine

Snack

Graham crackers	2
Peach	one medium (fresh, cooked or canned)

DAY ELEVEN

Breakfast

Orange	1 small
Cereal	cooked (Cream of Wheat) ½ cup with two tsp. sugar
Skim milk	one cup
Bread (toast)	one slice
Special margarine	one teaspoon

Lunch

Sandwich of:
  Smoked whitefish   3 ounces
  Bread   2 slices
  Special mayonnaise   1 tsp.
Salad of:
  Lettuce and greens
  Salad dressing of 2 teaspoons
    oil; salt, pepper, vinegar to
    taste
Applesauce   one-half cup with 1 tsp of sugar

Dinner

Macaroni casserole	1 cup
Meat for casserole	3 ounces beef, lamb, or pork
Spinach	one-half cup
Squash, winter	one-half cup with 1 tsp. brown sugar, 1 tsp. oil
Special margarine	2 tsp.
Skim milk	1 cup
Cantalope	one-fourth (or if frozen six pieces)
Sugar	1 tsp. or one glass of dry wine

Snack

Cream mints	4
Blueberries	three-fourths cup

DAY TWELVE

Breakfast

Banana	one-half small
Cereal	dry, prepared ¾ cup with 2 tsp sugar
Skim milk	1 cup
Bread (toast)	1 slice
Special margarine	1 teaspoon

Lunch

Sandwich of:	
Fried egg	with 2 tsp. of oil
Bread	2 slices
Special mayonnaise	1 tsp.
Salad of:	
Lettuce and tomatoes	
Salad dressing with no oil, salt, pepper and vinegar to taste; and one tsp. of sugar	
Raspberries	1 cup

Dinner

Swordfish steak	3 ounces (with tsp. of oil)
Hard roll	1 2-inch diameter
Cauliflower	one cup
Peas, green	one-half cup
Potato	one small, mashed with 1 tsp. oil
Skim milk	one cup
Pear	one small, fresh, cooked or canned
Sugar	2 tsp. or 2 glasses white wine

Snack

Saltines	5
Banana	one-half small

DAY THIRTEEN

Breakfast

Grapefruit Juice	1 small (4 ounce) glass)
Cereal	dry, prepared ¾ cup with 2 tsp. sugar
Skim milk	1 cup
Bread (toast)	1 slice
Special margarine	1 tsp.

Lunch

Beef bouillon	1 cup, clear
Cottage cheese	¾ cup, preferably uncreamed
Orange and grapefruit slices	one-half cup
Special mayonnaise	2 tsp.
Lettuce and watercress	
Hard roll	one large, 3-inch diameter
Special margarine	2 tsp.

Dinner

Ham, lean and trim	3 ounces
Dinner roll	1 2-inch diameter
Special margarine	2 tsp.
Asparagus	one cup
Corn, sweet	two-thirds cup (fresh or canned)
Skim milk	one cup
Apple	one small 2-inch diameter

Snack

Graham crackers	2
Honey	2 tsp.
Orange	1 small

THE FOURTEENTH DAY

Another day off! But this time you did not enter it with the spirit of a man about to compete with Henry the Eighth.

Also, if you are mathematically inclined, you may have some questions that deserve answers. Why is it, according to this book's own figures, that not every day's diet adds up to exactly 1800 calories? In reflection you can find a few spots where this diet shortchanged you—had you eating only 1773 calories, for example.

But what were you really cheated out of? A few fat and sugar calories—nothing you really needed. Also, the diet has not been too hard to follow at this level, has it? Perhaps no dramatic results, but certainly steady improvement—and a chance to learn how really to eat right.

If you want more spectacular results, this would be a good time to go back to the 1200 calorie diet. With two weeks behind you, it won't be too hard on your system—or psyche.

However, since most of us are starting to burn off a few pounds with the exercises, the jump rope and the walking/ running—let's figure that the best thing to do would be to put in another week on the 1800 calorie schedule.

Here it is—

Modified Fatty Acid Diet Values   1800 Calories

DAY FIFTEEN

Breakfast

Orange Juice	1 small (4 ounce) glass
Cereal	Oatmeal, cooked, ½ cup with 2 tsp. sugar
Skim milk	1 cup
Bread (toast)	1 slice
Special margarine	1 tsp.

Lunch

Sandwich of:

Turkey	3 ounces
Bread	2 slices
Special Mayonnaise	1 tsp.

Salad of:

Lettuce, celery, green pepper

Salad dressing	2 tsp. oil, salt, pepper, vinegar to taste
Pineapple	one-half cup with 1 tsp. sugar

Dinner

Whitefish	3 ounces breaded and fried in 2 tsp. oil
Spinach	one-half cup
Beets	one-half cup
Potato	1 small mashed with 1 tsp. oil
Hard roll	1 2-inch if fish is not breaded
Mayonnaise	2 tsp. mixed with relish to taste for tartar sauce
Skim milk	1 cup
Pear	1 small, fresh, cooked or canned
Sugar	2 tsp. or two 4 ounce glasses of white, dry wine

Snack

Soda crackers	3
Apple	1 small

DAY SIXTEEN

Breakfast

Grapefruit	one-half with 1 tsp. sugar
Cereal	Dry, prepared ¾ cup with 2 tsp. sugar
Skim milk	1 cup
Bread (toast)	1 slice
Special margarine	1 tsp.

Lunch

Sandwich of:	
Shrimp	3 ounces
Bread	2 slices
Special mayonnaise	1 tsp.
Salad of:	
Hearts of lettuce	
Salad dressing	2 tsp. of oil, salt, pepper and vinegar
Raisins	2 tablespoons full

Dinner

Veal	3 ounces with 2 ounces oil, and a stuffing of
Bread	1 slice
Peas, green	one-half cup
Eggplant	one-half to one cup
Potato	1 small mashed with 1 tsp. oil
Special margarine	2 tsp.
Skim milk	one cup
Cherries	10 large fresh, canned or cooked
Sugar	2 tsp.

Snack

Saltines	3
Plums	2 fresh, cooked or canned

DAY SEVENTEEN

Breakfast

Orange	1 small
Cereal	¾ cup dry prepared with 2 tsp. sugar
Skim milk	one cup
Bread (toast)	1 slice
Special margarine	1 tsp.

Lunch

Spaghetti	1 cup
Meatless sauce	¼ cup with 2 tsp. of oil
Salad of:	
Mixed greens: lettuce, celery, radishes, green peppers	
Salad dressing	2 tsp. of oil, salt, pepper and vinegar
Applesauce	½ cup

Dinner

Ground beef	3 ounces
Hard roll	1 2-inch diameter
Special margarine	2 teaspoons
Carrots	½ cup with 1 tsp. brown sugar
Broccoli	½ cup
Potato	1 small mashed in oil
Skim milk	1 cup
Peach	1 medium fresh, cooked or canned
Sugar	2 tsp.

Snack

Graham crackers	2
Banana	1 small

DAY EIGHTEEN

Breakfast

Grapefruit	one-half with 1 tsp. sugar
Cereal	Cream of Wheat ½ cup with 2 tsp. sugar
Skim milk	one cup
Bread (toast)	1 slice
Special margarine	1 tsp.

Lunch

Sandwich of:	
Chicken	3 ounces
Bread	2 slices
Special mayonnaise	1 tsp.
Salad of:	
Apple, raisins and lettuce	one serving with 2 tsp. mayonnaise

Dinner

Halibut steak	3 ounces with 2 tsp. oil
Dinner roll	1 2-inch diameter (or use for breading fish)
Asparagus	one-half to one cup
Cauliflower	one cup
Potatoes, sweet	¼ cup mashed with 1 tsp. oil
Special margarine	2 tsp.
Skim milk	one cup
Figs	2 large, fresh or canned or dried
Sugar	2 tsp.

Snack

Soda crackers	3
Tangerine	1 large, fresh or preserved

DAY NINETEEN

Breakfast

Banana	1 small
Cereal	Dry, prepared ¾ cup with 2 tsp. sugar
Skim milk	1 cup
Bread (toast)	1 slice
Special margarine	1 tsp.

Lunch

Sandwich of:

Smoked whitefish	3 ounces
Bread	2 slices
Special mayonnaise	1 tsp.

Salad of:

Watercress, escarole and lettuce	
Salad dressing	2 tsp. oil, plus salt, pepper and vinegar
Strawberries	1 cup

Dinner

Noodles	1 cup cooked with
Tuna fish	3 ounces and 2 ounces of oil, if desired. Casserole or creamed.
Peas, green	one-half cup
Cauliflower	one cup
Special margarine	2 tsp.
Skim milk	one cup
sugar	2 tsp. or 2 glasses wine
Orange	1 small

Snack

Graham crackers	2
Apple	1 small 2-inch diameter

DAY TWENTY
Breakfast

Orange Juice	1 small (4 ounce) glass
Cereal	Oatmeal ½ cup cooked with 2 tsp. sugar
Skim milk	1 cup
Bread (toast)	1 slice
Special margarine	1 tsp.

Lunch

Sandwich of:

Egg	1 boiled, and chopped for egg salad
Bread	2 slices
Mayonnaise	2 tsp. mustard and season to taste

Salad of:
Lettuce and tomatoes
Salad dressing of one tsp. of
oil, salt, pepper, vinegar

Grape Juice	1 small (4 ounce) glass

Dinner

Roast Beef	3 ounces well trimmed, no gravy or pot liquor!
Cornbread	one and ¼-inch cubes
Mushrooms	one-half cup
Peas, green	one-half cup
Potato	1 small mashed in 1 tsp. oil
Special margarine	2 tsp.
Skim milk	1 cup
Cantalope	¼ or if frozen 6 pieces
Sugar	2 tsp. or 2 glasses wine, dry— red or white

Snack

Saltines	3
Banana	1 small

THE TWENTY-FIRST DAY

Another day off, and by this time you are beginning to prove to yourself the benefits of this diet. You look better, your head is cleared, and your friends—especially the fat ones —are beginning to try to tempt you.

You see, we live in a world of organization men, and they do hate to see anyone getting out of step. "Go ahead, Charlie," they love to taunt us, "have a bit more"—a bit more strudel, booze, or whatever is lying around at the time.

Go ahead—but only if you want to eat yourself to death.

Don't listen to them. A few weeks from now, they will beg you to tell them how you did it. Social pressures, like most other things, are all right in their place and time, but as your health and appearance improve, others will want to follow *your* example.

Nor are you starting out on this path alone. This is a national, as well as a personal problem—and it is receiving national attention. You know that you can't take it with you; but why not stay here a while longer and use it, even if you do have to pay taxes on it?

CONTINUING BENEFITS—FOR THE REST OF YOUR LIFE

Incidentally, the final week of this diet is not the last week you should use it. These final six diets are going to yield about 2400 calories. This should give you continued weight control, with satisfying meals, for the rest of your life.

However, many of us will put on weight eating 2400 calories; so for such people a 2,400 calorie diet can be too much—particularly for those under five feet, five inches.

Therefore, regulate the diet to *your* size, *your* activities, *your* age.

For example, as we grow older, our body usually slows down and needs less food. A man of 65 needs about 10% less calories than an equally active man of 45. When we're 25 we need about 10% more food than at 45. The same, of course, holds true for women. Therefore, eat your age.

Once appetites are retrained, these diets should add up to adequate, enjoyable meals that we can comfortably follow the rest of our days. Start now to form the habits of eating wisely—and well.

Modified Fatty Acid Diets   2400 Calories

DAY TWENTY-ONE

Breakfast

Grapefruit	½ with 2 tsp. sugar
Cereal	¾ cup dry with 2 tsp. sugar
Skim milk	1 cup
Bread (toast)	1 slice
Jelly, jam	1 tsp.
Special Margarine	1 tsp.

Lunch

Sandwich of:

Chicken	3 ounces
Bread	2 slices
Special mayonnaise	1 tsp.

Salad of:
Lettuce and mixed greens
Salad dressing of 1 tablespoon oil, salt, pepper,
vinegar

Baked Apple	Small with 1 tsp. sugar

Dinner

Haddock	4 ounces fried in 1 tablespoon of oil
Bread	1 slice may be used to bread fish
Spinach	½ cup
Carrots	½ cup with 1 tsp. brown or white sugar
Potato	1 small mashed in 1 tsp. oil
Special margarine	2 tsp.

Mayonnaise	1 tablespoon with relish to taste for tartar sauce
Skim milk	1 cup
Pear	1 small, cooked, canned or fresh
Sugar	2 tsp.

Snack

Bread—cinnamon toast with sugar	2 slices 2 tsp.
Special margarine or oil	2 tsp.
Orange juice	1 small (4 ounce) glass
Banana	½ small

DAY TWENTY-TWO

Breakfast

Orange Juice	1 small (4 ounce) glass
Cereal	Oatmeal ½ cup with 2 tsp. sugar
Skim milk	1 cup
Bread (toast)	1 slice
Jam, jelly	1 tsp.
Special margarine	1 tsp.

Lunch

Chicken salad	3 ounces chicken
Bread	2 slices
Special mayonnaise	1 tsp.
Salad of:	
Mixed greens	
Salad dressing	1 tablespoon oil, salt, pepper, vinegar
Strawberries	1 cup with 1 tsp. sugar

Dinner

Veal	4 ounces with 1 tablespoon oil
Bread	one slice as dressing for veal
Cauliflower	1 cup
Peas, green	½ cup
Potato	1 small mashed in 1 tsp. oil
Skim milk	1 cup
Mayonnaise	1 tablespoon
Margarine	2 tsp.
Sugar	2 tsp.
Plums	2 medium fresh, cooked or canned

Snack

Soda crackers	6
Honey	2 tsp.
Special margarine	2 tsp.
Pear	one small fresh, cooked or canned

DAY TWENTY-THREE

Breakfast

Orange	1 small
Cereal	¾ cup dry with 2 tsp. sugar
Skim milk	1 cup
Bread (toast)	1 slice
Jam, jelly	1 tsp.
Special margarine	1 tsp.

Lunch

Rice	1 cup
Lobster pieces	2 ounces
Oil for preparation	2 tsp.
Salad of:	
Grated carrots and raisins	one serving with
Special mayonnaise	2 tsp.

Dinner

Lamb chop	4 ounces with 1 tablespoon oil
Hard roll	1 2-inch diameter
Special margarine	2 tsp.
Asparagus	½ cup
Beets	½ cup
Special mayonnaise	1 tablespoon
Skim milk	1 cup
Raspberries	1 cup
Sugar	3 tsp.

Snack

Graham crackers	4
Marshmallows	2
Dates	4

DAY TWENTY-FOUR

Breakfast

Peach	one medium with 2 tsp. sugar
Cereal	Dry, prepared ¾ oz. with 2 tsp. sugar
Bread (toast)	1 slice
Skim milk	1 cup
Special margarine	1 tsp.
Marmalade	1 tsp.

Lunch

Sandwich of:	
Smoked turkey	3 ounces
Bread	2 slices
Special mayonnaise	1 tsp.
Salad of:	
Mixed greens	
Salad dressing	1 tablespoon oil or 1½ tablespoons of French dressing
Applesauce	½ cup

Dinner

Beef steak	4 ounces trimmed of fat and broiled
Spinach with mushrooms	½ cup
Carrots	½ cup with 1 teaspoon sugar, brown or white
Potato	1 small mashed with 1 tsp. oil
Mayonnaise, special	2 tsp.
Skim milk	1 cup
Apricots	2 medium fresh or dried
Sugar	2 tsp.

Snack

Saltines	10
Sugar	2 tsp.
Special margarine	2 tsp.
Raisins	2 tablespoons full

DAY TWENTY-FIVE

Breakfast

Blueberries	⅔ cup with 2 tsp. sugar
Pancakes	3 thin 4-inch in diameter or 1 waffle
Skim milk	1 cup
Special margarine or oil	1 tsp.
Honey or syrup	2 ounces

Lunch

Sandwich of:	
Smoked salmon	3 ounces
Bread	2 slices
Cream cheese	1 tsp. Onion if desired
Salad of:	
Lettuce and tomatoes	
Salad dressing	2 tsp. of oil plus salt, pepper and vinegar
Peach	1 medium, fresh, cooked or canned

Dinner

Red snapper	4 ounces broiled in 1 tablespoon oil
Hard roll	1 2-inch diameter
Cabbage cooked or as cole slaw	1 cup
Special mayonnaise	1 tablespoon
Green peas	½ cup
Potato	1 small mashed with 1 tsp. of oil
Skim milk	1 cup
Orange	1 small
Sugar	3 tsp.

Snack

Graham crackers	4
Jam	1 tsp.
Special margarine	2 tsp.
Pineapple	½ cup

DAY TWENTY-SIX

Breakfast

Grapefruit Juice	1 small (4 ounce) glass with 1 tsp. sugar
Cereal	¾ cup dry, prepared with 2 tsp. sugar
Skim milk	1 cup
Bread (toast)	1 slice
Jam, jelly	1 tsp.
Special margarine	1 tsp.

Lunch

Sandwich of:

Chicken	3 ounces
Bread	2 slices
Special mayonnaise	1 tsp.

Salad of:
Cucumbers and tomatoes
With salad dressing of 1 tablespoon of oil, plus salt, pepper and vinegar to taste

Strawberries	1 cup

Dinner

Canadian bacon	2 ounces
Eggs	2 for Eggs Benedict
Muffin for above	1 3-inch in diameter
Asparagus	1 cup
Mayonnaise	1 tablespoon for sauce
Green peas	½ cup
Potato	1 small mashed with 1 tsp. oil
Skim milk	1 cup
Grapes	12 fresh or preserved
Special margarine	2 tsp.

Snack

Bread—cinnamon toast with	2 slices
sugar	2 tsp.
and oil or special margarine	2 tsp.
Orange Juice	1 cup (8 ounces)

FOOD EXCHANGE LISTS

Sometimes you will wish to vary the diets, and substitute one food for another. These Exchange Lists will show you how to do this. Simply substitute one food within each list for another food within the same list. For example, you may substitute one-half a small grapefruit for ten large cherries. Or one-half cup of spaghetti for one slice of bread.

You may also substitute vegetables for fruits, or fruits for vegetables. But do not substitute the meat, fat, milk or bread foods for each other. To take an extra slice of meat, for example, instead of a slice of bread, would throw off your diet. Substitute meat only for meat, milk only for milk, fat only for fat, and bread only for other carbohydrates in List 4.

Eggs may be substituted only for the meat exchanges in List 5.

By using these lists, you will give your meals great variety and flavor, and at the same time keep perfectly within the limits of your diet.

FOOD EXCHANGE LISTS

Milk Exchanges—List 1

Nonfat Dried Milk	¼ Cup
Skim Milk	1 Cup
Buttermilk (Made from skim milk)	1 Cup

Vegetables Exchanges—List 2

Vegetable A As desired

Asparagus	Cauliflower
Beans, String, Young	Celery
Broccoli	Chicory
Brussels Sprouts	Cucumber
Cabbage	Escarole
Lettuce	Eggplant
Mushrooms	Sauerkraut
Okra	Squash, summer
Radishes	Tomatoes
Pepper	Watercress

"Greens"

Beet Greens	Kale
Chard, Swiss	Mustard Greens
Collard	Spinach
Dandelion Greens	Turnip Greens

Vegetable B
   (½ cup per serving)

Beets	Pumpkin
Carrots	Rutabaga
Onions	Squash, Winter
Peas, Green	Turnip

Fruit Exchanges—List 3

Apple (2-inch diam)	1
Applesauce	½ cup

Apricots	
Fresh	2 medium
Dried	4 halves
Banana	½ small
Blackberries	1 cup
Blueberries	⅔ cup
Cantaloupe (6-inch diam)	¼
Cherries	10 large
Dates	2
Figs	
Fresh	2 Large
Dried	2
Grape Juice	½ Cup
Grapefruit Juice	½ Cup
Grapefruit	½ Small
Grapes	12
Honeydew melon (7-inch diam)	⅛ Small
Mango	½ Small
Orange	1 Small
Orange Juice	½ Cup
Papaya	⅓ Medium
Peach	1 Small
Pear	1 Small
Pineapple	½ Cup
Pineapple Juice	⅓ Cup
Plums	2 medium
Prunes, Dried	2 medium
Raisins	2 tbsp.
Raspberries	1 Cup
Strawberries	1 Cup
Tangerine	1 Large
Watermelon	1 Cup

Bread Exchanges—List 4

Bread	1 Slice
* Biscuit Muffin, Roll (2-inch)	1

* Cornbread (1½-inch cube)	1
Sherbet	1 tbsp.
Carbonated beverages	2 oz.
Cereal, Cooked	⅓ Cup
Dry, Flakes, Puffed	¾ Cup
Rice, grits, Cooked	½ Cup
Spaghetti, Noodles, Cooked	½ Cup
Macaroni, etc., Cooked	½ Cup
Crackers, Graham	2
Saltine	5
Soda	3
Beans, Peas, Dried, Cooked	½ Cup
Corn, Sweet	⅓ Cup
Corn on Cob (Medium Ear)	½
Potatoes, White (2-inch dia.)	1
Potatoes, Sweet	¼ Cup
Parsnips	⅔ Cup

Meat, Fish, and Poultry Exchanges—List 5

Select meat from this group for 3 meals a week:

Beef, eye of round, top and bottom round, lean ground round, lean rump, tenderloin	1 oz.
Lamb, Leg only	1 oz.
Pork, Lean Loin	1 oz.
Ham, Lean and well trimmed	1 oz.

Make selections from this group for 11 meals a week:

Chicken, no skin	1 oz.
Turkey, no skin	1 oz.
Veal	1 oz.
Fish	1 oz.
Shellfish	1 oz.
Meat substitute, cottage cheese, preferably uncreamed	¼ Cup

* Made with corn or cottonseed oil. Diets planned according to ADA Exchange System. Meat exchanges were calculated as containing 3 gm. fat instead of ADA value of 5 gm.

Eggs—List 6

Four eggs per week allowed in each diet plan as a substitute for one No. 5 exchange.

Fat Exchange—List 7

50% Polyunsaturated

Corn Oil	1 tsp.
Cottonseed Oil	1 tsp.
Safflower Oil	1 tsp.

Mayonnaise made with corn or
cottonseed oil   1 tsp.

French Dressing made with
corn or cottonseed oil   2 tsp.

30%-40% polyunsaturated

Special margarines	1 tsp.
Special shortenings	1 tsp.

** *Sugar Exchange—List 8*

White, Brown or Maple Sugar	1 tsp.
Corn, Syrup, Honey, Molasses	1 tsp.
Candy (no chocolate)	
Gum drop	1 medium or 6 small
Hard type	6-8 small fruit drops
Mints, Cream	3-4
Marshmallow, Plain	1 average
Jelly, Jams, all varieties	1 tbsp.
Sherbet	1 tbsp.
Carbonated Beverages	2 oz.

Modified Fatty Acid Diet Values   1800 Calories

	B	L	D	S
Milk, Skim	1 X			
Vegetables "A"		Ad Lib	Ad Lib	

** 1/2 oz. alcohol = 1 sugar exchange and may be substituted at discretion of physician.

			1 X	
Vegetables "B"				
Fruit	1 X	1 X	1 X	2 X
Bread and Cereals	2 X	2 X	1 X	1 X
Meat, Fish and Poultry		3 X	3 X	
Fats	1 X	3 X	5 X	
Sweets and Sugar	3 X	3 X	3 X	

To Reduce 1800 Calories to 1200 Calories

Breakfast:

No toast, oil, special mayonnaise or sugar.

Lunch:

No sugar.
Reduce amount of chicken to 2 oz.

Dinner:

No potato with oil.

Snack:

None.

Exchanges:

Milk	No change
Vegetable	No change
Fruit	Subtract 2 exchanges
Bread and cereals	Subtract 2 exchanges
Meat, Fish, Poultry	Subtract 1 exchange
Fat	Subtract 3 exchanges
Sweet, sugar	Subtract all exchange

To Increase 1800 Calories to 2400 Calories

Breakfast:

Add jelly to toast	1 teaspoon
Add sugar to grapefruit	1 teaspoon

Lunch:

Increase oil in dressing to	1 tablespoon

Dinner:

Haddock)	4 oz.
Breaded)	1 slice
Fried in oil)	1 tablespoon
Mayonnaise in relish	1 tablespoon
Margarine—special	2 teaspoons

Snack:

Bread—Cinnamon Toast)	2 slices
With Sugar)	2 teaspoons
Oil	2 teaspoons
Orange Juice	½ cup
Banana	½ small

Exchanges:

Milk	No Change
Vegetables	No Change
Fruit	No Change
Bread and Cereals	Add 1 Exchange
Meat, Fish, Poultry	Add 1 Exchange
Fat	Add 9 Exchanges—3 may be special mayonnaise
Sweets and Sugar	Add 3 Exchanges

Chapter Fourteen

YOUR HEALTH AUDIT EXAMINATIONS

Various corporate and insurance groups have been conducting health audit examinations over the years and analyzing the results. Their experience has shown that many of the more prolonged, complicated and expensive examinations yield very little in the way of diagnostic information. On the other hand, some simple and quick laboratory tests are very rich in their return of positive information.

Based on this information, the examinations which you should follow fall into two groups, A and B, outlined below.

AN "A" EXAMINATION MAY INCLUDE ALL OF THE FOLLOWING:

> Medical history
> Physical examination
> Rectal digital examination
> Cervical smear and "Pap" test
> Complete blood count
> Urinalysis

Blood Chemistries:
  Sugar
  Nitrogen
  Protein
Proctoscopic Examination
Electrocardiogram
Chest X-ray
Feces Examination

A "B" EXAMINATION MAY INCLUDE ALL OF THE FOLLOWING

Medical history
Physical examination
Rectal digital examination
Cervical smear and "Pap" test
Complete blood count
Urinalysis
Blood chemistries:
  Sugar
  Nitrogen
  Protein
Feces examination

In order to obtain maximum usefulness of the preventative features of this plan, the following program is suggested:

Anyone from age 20 to 30—one "A" exam and one "B" exam should be done on an alternate 18 to 24 months.

From 30 to 40 the same alternating of "A" and "B" exams should occur, but on a 12 to 18 month schedule.

From 40 or 45 on, an "A" exam should be done annually.

HISTORY AND PHYSICAL CONDITION QUESTIONNAIRE

The descriptions here of the "A" and "B" examinations are not meant to imply that each and every exam must be done in a mechanical and impersonal fashion; but rather that such a procedure will yield a maximum amount of information within financial reason.

In addition, historical and physical information are both necessary to complete each examination. A form of questionnaire history is included here to be checked off by you before going to your physician.

HEALTH AUDIT QUESTIONNAIRE

NAME_____

PERSONAL MEDICAL HISTORY

	: Check : : Mark :	At what age?
Chickenpox	: :	
Measles	: :	
German Measles	: :	
Smallpox	: :	
Diphtheria	: :	
Whooping Cough	: :	
Scarlet Fever	: :	
Influenza	: :	
Pneumonia	: :	
Rheumatic Fever	: :	
Nephritis	: :	
Malaria	: :	
Typhoid Fever	: :	
Tonsillitis	: :	
Tuberculosis	: :	
Venereal: (Syphilis)	: :	
(gonorrhea)	: :	
Epilepsy	: :	
Serious Injuries	: :	
Diabetes	: :	
Allergies	: :	
(As hay fever, asthma, hives)	:	
Exposure to T.B.	: :	

LIST DRUG OR FOOD ALLERGIES:

1)_____
2)_____
3)_____
4)_____

SURGERY AND AGE AT TIME:

1)_____ _____
2)_____ _____
3)_____ _____
4)_____ _____

DO ANY OF THE FOLLOWING DISEASES OCCUR IN YOUR FAMILY?*

	Yes	No
High Blood Pressure?*	____	____
Diabetes?	____	____
Heart Disease?	____	____
Kidney Disease?	____	____
Cancer?	____	____
Blood Disease?	____	____
Tuberculosis?	____	____
Allergies? (hay fever, asthma, hives)	____	____
Migraine?	____	____

*note: FAMILY refers to blood relatives.

FAMILY* HISTORY

*note: FAMILY refers to blood relatives.

IF LIVING

	: Age :	: State of : : Health :	Any present Illness?
Father	:	:	:
Mother	:	:	:
Brothers	:	:	:
	:	:	:
	:	:	:
	:	:	:
Sisters	:	:	:
	:	:	:
	:	:	:
	:	:	:

IF DEAD

	: Age at : : Death :	Cause
Father	:	
Mother	:	
Brothers	:	
	:	
	:	
	:	
Sisters	:	
	:	
	:	
	:	

	Yes	No
Does stomach trouble occur in your family?	____	____
Rheumatism or arthritis?	____	____
Headaches?	____	____
Has anyone in your family ever had fits or convulsions? (epilepsy)?	____	____
Nervous exhaustion or nervousness occur in your family?	____	____
Do you come from a sickly family?	____	____
Did anyone in your family ever have a nervous breakdown or need to be a patient in a mental hospital?	____	____

HABITS

ERAGE Amounts of: Tobacco___Kind and amount per day_____

Alcohol___Amount per day or week_____

Coffee___No. of cups per day_____

Tension and emotional stress___   Less than average_____

in your work: Average_____

More than average_____

Very heavy_____

If you *can* answer YES to the question asked, put a circle around the Yes.
If you have to answer NO to the question asked, put a circle around the No.
ANSWER all questions. If you are not sure, guess. Answer the questions literally, paying particular attention
to the objectives such as *always, often, frequently, never*, etc.

1.	Do you use glasses to read? Is your vision defective?	Yes	No
2.	Do you *need* glasses to see things at a distance?	Yes	No
3.	Has your eyesight *ever* blacked out completely?	Yes	No
4.	Do your eyes *continually* blink or water?	Yes	No
5.	Do you *often* have bad pains in your eyes?	Yes	No
6.	Are your eyes *often* red or inflamed?	Yes	No
7.	Are you hard of hearing or have constant noise in your head?	Yes	No
8.	Have you *ever* had a bad running ear?	Yes	No
9.	Are you *often* troubled with bad spells of sneezing?	Yes	No
10.	Is your nose *continually* stuffed up or running?	Yes	No
11.	Have you at times had *bad* nose bleeds?	Yes	No
12.	Do you have more than 4 colds a year?	Yes	No
13.	When you catch a cold, do you *always* have to go to bed?	Yes	No
14.	Are you troubled by *constant* coughing?	Yes	No
15.	Have you *ever* coughed up blood?	Yes	No
16.	Do you *sometimes* have severe soaking sweats at night?	Yes	No
17.	Have you ever had a chronic chest condition?	Yes	No
18.	Have you ever had T.B. (Tuberculosis)?	Yes	No
19.	Did you ever live with anyone who had T.B.?	Yes	No
20.	Has a doctor *ever* said your blood pressure was too high?	Yes	No
21.	Has a doctor *ever* said your blood pressure was too low?	Yes	No
22.	Do you *ever* have pains in the heart or chest?	Yes	No
23.	Are you *often* bothered by thumping of the heart?	Yes	No
24.	Does your heart *often* race like mad?	Yes	No
25.	Do you *often* have difficulty in breathing?	Yes	No
26.	Do you get out of breath *long before* anyone else?	Yes	No
27.	Do you *sometimes* get out of breath just sitting still?	Yes	No
28.	Are your ankles *often* badly swollen?	Yes	No
29.	Do you suffer from frequent cramps in your legs when resting?	Yes	No
30.	Do you get leg cramps or pains while walking?	Yes	No
31.	Do you usually use more than 1 pillow at night?	Yes	No

D

32. Have you lost more than half your teeth?... Yes
33. Are you troubled by bleeding gums?.. Yes
34. Have you *often* had severe toothaches?.. Yes
35. Do you have a sore tongue at times?.. Yes
36. Is your appetite *always* poor?.. Yes
37. Do you *sometimes* have trouble swallowing?... Yes
38. Do you *often* suffer from an upset stomach, or indigestion?........................ Yes
39. Do you *frequently* feel bloated, or belch a lot after eating? .... Yes
40. Do you *often* have spells of nausea or vomiting?..................................... Yes
41. Do severe pains in the stomach *often* double you up? .... Yes
42. Has a doctor *ever* said you had stomach ulcers?..................................... Yes
43. Do you suffer from *frequent* loose bowel movements? .... Yes
44. Have you *ever* had severe bloody diarrhea?.. Yes
45. Were you *ever* troubled with intestinal worms?.. Yes
46. Do you constantly suffer from bad constipation?.. Yes
47. Have you *ever* had piles (rectal hemorrhoids)?....................................... Yes
48. Have you *ever* had jaundice or serious liver or gall bladder trouble?........... Yes
49. Have you had severe anemia?.. Yes
50. Have you had a tumor or cancer?... Yes
51. Are you definitely underweight, or overweight?... Yes
52. Are there foods you cannot eat?... Yes
53. Have you *ever* had tarry black bowel movements?.................................... Yes

E

54. Are your joints often painfully swollen?... Yes
55. Do your muscles and joints constantly feel stiff?....................................... Yes
56. Are you crippled with severe rheumatism (arthritis)? .... Yes
57. Do weak or painful feet bother you?... Yes
58. Do pains in the back make it hard for you to keep up with your work?.......... Yes
59. Are you troubled with a serious disability or deformity? .... Yes

F

60. Is your skin very sensitive or tender?.. Yes
61. Do cuts in your skin usually stay open a long time?................................... Yes
62. Does your skin often break out in a rash?.. Yes
63. Are you often bothered by severe itching?... Yes
64. Are you often troubled with boils?.. Yes

G

65. Do you suffer badly from frequent severe headaches? .... Yes
66. Do you *frequently* feel faint or have spells of severe dizziness? .... Yes
67. Have you fainted more than twice in your life?.. Yes
68. Do you have constant numbness or tingling in any part of your body?.......... Yes
69. Was any part of your body ever paralyzed?.. Yes
70. Were you ever knocked unconscious?.. Yes
71. Have you ever had a twitching of face, head or shoulders? .... Yes
72. Did you ever have a fit or convulsion (epilepsy)?..................................... Yes

H

73. Have you ever had anything wrong with your genitals (privates)? .... Yes
74. Are your genitals *often* painful or sore?.. Yes
75. Has a doctor *ever* said you had a hernia (rupture)? .... Yes
76. Have you *ever* passed blood while urinating (passing water)? .... Yes
77. Do you have trouble starting your stream when urinating? .... Yes
78. Do you have to get up every night and urinate?... Yes
79. During the day, do you *usually* have to urinate frequently? .... Yes
80. Do you *often* have severe burning pain when you urinate? .... Yes
81. Do you sometimes lose control of your bladder?.. Yes
82. Has a doctor *ever* said you had kidney or bladder disease? .... Yes

3. Do you *often* get spells of complete exhaustion or fatigue? .... Yes   No
4. Does working tire you out *completely?*.. Yes   No
5. Do you *usually* get up tired and exhausted in the morning? .... Yes   No
5. Does every little effort wear you out?... Yes   No
7. Are you *constantly* too tired and exhausted even to eat? .... Yes   No

3. Are you frequently ill or confined to bed by illness? .... Yes   No
9. Are you always in poor health or considered a sickly person? .... Yes   No
). Do severe pains and aches make it impossible for you to do your work?.................... Yes   No
4. Do you wear yourself out worrying about your health? .... Yes   No
2. Are you *constantly* made miserable by poor health? .... Yes   No
4. Are you *especially* concerned about cancer or heart disease? .... Yes   No

4. Do cold hands or feet trouble you even in hot weather? .... Yes   No
5. Do you usually eat sweets or other food between meals? .... Yes   No
   Does your face often get badly flushed?.. Yes   No
7. Do you sweat a great deal even in cold weather?.. Yes   No
3. Do you have hot or cold spells?.. Yes   No
9. Do you bite your nails badly? .... Yes   No
). Are you troubled by stuttering or stammering?... Yes   No
1. Are you a sleep walker or a bed wetter?.. Yes   No
2. Were you a bed wetter between the ages of 8 and 14? .... Yes   No

5. Do you usually have great difficulty in falling asleep or staying asleep?..................... Yes   No
6. Do you get adequate regular rest (6 to 8 hours in 24)? .... Yes   No

   Do you sweat or tremble a lot during examinations or questioning, or when approached by a   Yes   No
   superior?   .... Yes   No
3. Does your work fall to pieces when the boss or a superior is watching you?............... Yes   No
7. Does your thinking get completely mixed up when you have to do things quickly?........ Yes   No
   Must you do things very slowly in order to do them without mistakes?.................... Yes   No
9. Do you frequently get directions and orders wrong? .... Yes   No
   Do strange people or places make you afraid?.. Yes   No
   Are you scared to be alone or among strangers? .... Yes   No
2. Is it always hard for you to make up your mind? .... Yes   No
   Do you wish you always had someone at your side to advise you?........................... Yes   No
   Are you considered a clumsy person?... Yes   No
   Does it bother you to eat anywhere except in your own home?................................ Yes   No

   Do you feel alone and sad at a party?... Yes   No
   Do you usually feel unhappy and depressed or cry often? .... Yes   No
   Are you always miserable and blue or does life look hopeless? .... Yes   No
   Do you often wish you were dead and away from it all?...... .... Yes   No

   Does worrying get you down? Does worrying run in your family?............................ Yes   No
   Are you considered a nervous person?.. Yes   No
   Did you ever have a nervous breakdown?.. Yes   No
   Were you ever a patient in a mental hospital (for your nerves)?............................. Yes   No

   Are you extremely shy or sensitive?.. Yes   No
   Do you come from a shy or sensitive family?.. Yes   No
   Do your feelings easily hurt? Does criticism always upset you?.............................. Yes   No
   Are you considered a touchy person?... Yes   No
   Do people usually misunderstand you?......... .... Yes   No

Q

129. Do you have to be on your guard even with friends? .... Yes
130. Do you usually do things on sudden impulse? .... Yes
131. Do you go to pieces if you don't constantly control yourself? .... Yes
132. Do little annoyances get on your nerves and make you irritated? .... Yes
133. Does it make you angry to have anyone tell you what to do? .... Yes
134. Do people often annoy and irritate you? .... Yes
135. Do you flare up in anger if you can't have what you want right away? .... Yes
136. Do you often get into a violent rage? .... Yes

R

137. Do you often shake or tremble? .... Yes
138. Are you constantly keyed up and jittery? .... Yes
139. Do sudden noises make you jump or shake badly? .... Yes
140. Do you tremble or feel weak whenever someone shouts at you? .... Yes
141. Do you become scared at sudden movements or noises at night? .... Yes
142. Are you often awakened out of your sleep by frightening dreams? .... Yes
143. Do frightening thoughts keep coming back in your mind? .... Yes
144. Do you often become suddenly scared for no good reason? .... Yes
145. Do you often break out in a cold sweat? .... Yes

Part Three

Longevity and Common Sense

Chapter Fifteen

FAD DIETS

It is hard to find any area where half as much contradictory advice is available as can be found on food. With such a profusion of information, we must too often expect to find ignorance rather than knowledge.

In evaluating this mass of material, there are two basic principles that must be remembered and applied if we are not to be driven to madness.

The first principle is that of suspended judgment. The final, true, correct answers on diet, and on health foods, haven't been discovered yet.

And, secondly, just as surely as these principles are discovered, they will not apply to everyone in the world. Fingerprints are different, footprints are different, and no two people's diet requirements are ever alike.

Therefore, remembering that one man's beneficial diet may be another man's certain poison, let's examine some of the most popular food theories of our day, and see what medical science has to say about each of them:

CALORIES DO COUNT

Probably the most popular new diet in circulation tells you to eat lots of fat and no starches, and, by this simple formula, lose weight.

This ketogenic diet (that is its proper medical name) is at least forty years old—and it can be useful when properly handled. At one time it was about the only way a diabetic could hope to keep on living. Before the use of phenobarbital and other drugs, it was frequently the remedy for epilepsy. Even today there are diseases which can be handled well by placing the patient on a high fat, low starch diet.

But none of these facts means that such a diet is simple, easy to eat, or to prescribe. Too many drawbacks in this diet make it unpopular with physicians.

The worst hazard is that of death. If the diet is followed to the letter, acidosis can occur at any time, and with acidosis, unless heroic medical measures are undertaken quickly, death occurs.

Another problem with this type of diet is water loss. In each of us, a great deal of weight is made up of water. A high fat, low starch diet dries most people up. On the scales, for the first four weeks, this looks great because the weight goes down. The problem comes when the dieter goes back on a balanced schedule of eating, for then the cells of the body are again able to hold the water they want, and the scales go bouncing back up.

WHAT ABOUT FASTING?

Have we all forgotten the great Mahatma Gandhi this quickly? Fasting as a way of life, as well as a trick of weight control is old, old, old. But today it is being sold as a great revelation in many publications.

Fasting was not invented in 1963, or in any other period of history. The situation—no food—is no different from being really poor.

In many parts of the world, for example, periods of starvation are still common. The long-lived Hunzingas are a dramatic example of this. In the Spring, as always within the memory of man, the food runs out. For some there may be a sustenance level of food left, but for many there is none. Yet these people are famous for virility and activity beyond their nineties and hundreds. Obviously this problem of three square meals a day is not solved in their mode of life—but their length of life looks far better than it does for the well fed.

All in all, there is nothing mysterious or occult about fasting. Most people in good health, under the age of sixty, can undertake a brief one to three day fast with safety. However, you would be foolish to try it without the advice of your physician.

Crash diets, of which fasting is the most dramatic, are usually neither permanent nor satisfactory ways to lose weight. Habits are not changed in moments, and the unexpressed hope of the crash diet is always that habits will be changed without effort. This is simply a case in which another form of wishful thinking is substituted for hard, cold logic.

THE ROLE OF OUR GLANDS

Those of us who continue in the deadly overweight pattern can find many excuses to justify our compulsive behavior. "It's my glands, Doctor," is a favorite complaint of many. Well, in a very few cases this statement may be true. And the fatter the person is—say, forty, fifty, sixty pounds over-weight—the more likely it is to be true.

But even here, overeating may have caused the very failure of these glands that lead to a never-ceasing spiral of more and more weight. Glands can only operate best when we are of normal size. The bigger we get, the harder they must work; and so, at some size and weight, our glands are going to be burdened beyond capacity.

For example, diabetes—one of today's commoner diseases is frequently found in the obese. This diabetic condition was caused by a gland failure. The pancreas, that organ which manufactures insulin, became exhausted by being too long overtaxed, and simply quit working.

Apparently this same problem of exhaustion can happen in other glands. As another example, the thyroid, which acts as the thermostat of our internal fires, may wear out and stop making its chemicals after too much overloading.

So, if you are extremely overweight, and you suspect that the cause is your glands, see your doctor. He is the one who can find out which gland it is, and do something about it. Otherwise, your excess weight is simply caused by simple overeating, and can be corrected by the plan we have sug-gested in this book.

HEREDITY AND YOUR WEIGHT

There are families of fatties, but this does not mean that fatness runs in the family. What it does mean is: in such a group, eating, as an end in itself, is being used as a substitute expression of love, reward, and attention.

Only a few of us live in such households. But all of us in the western world live in *nations* of fatties. Many of our signs of affection revolve around food. These habits are left over from days of short food supply. Now they serve only to add weight and take away life from many. It's up to each of us to find other ways to express affection that are not related to eat, eat, eat.

THE VEGETARIAN ROAD TO LONGEVITY

George Bernard Shaw, Mahatma Gandhi and Bernarr MacFadden would all be called food faddists by most of us. We know that they all reached old age in excellent health, with as much or more mental alertness at 75 than they showed in their early years. It would not be wise, in a study on longevity, to ignore their diets and thoughts on food; they all made crusades of their eating habits and attempted to get others to join them.

These men were, for most of their lives, vegetarians. Gandhi ate meat for a few years, but could never force himself to like the taste of it. The other two never touched meat during their adult life.

Mahatma Gandhi was undoubtedly the most famous person to fast in our times. He had fasted many times before he began to make political capital out of his refusal to eat—his mother had quite often fasted during his boyhood for religious reasons.

In the last days of his life, incidentally, during the riots which eventually saw Gandhi's assassination, the Mahatma said a most interesting thing. He stated with some prescience of his fate, "I don't think that I shall live to be 125." This comment seems strange to the western mind, which cannot accept such longevity as a natural goal. But it was in perfect keeping with the Indian experience, since many of them do live to such a great age.

There is nothing medically wrong with such a vegetarian

diet. But you and I enjoy the taste of well prepared meats, as much, if not more, than we enjoy a fine pastry. It may be possible to live out a great number of years in grand health as a vegetarian—but the road is probably too unpleasant a one for most of us to travel.

IN SUMMARY

As long as our diet is balanced in essentials—fats, carbohydrates, proteins—no great problems should arise.

Our bodies are wonderful mechanisms and they can manufacture nearly all the correct chemicals we need for good nutrition. They need only be given the proper raw materials from which to start production.

Chapter Sixteen

STRESS, SMOKING AND OTHER GOBLINS

There is a tremendous amount of misleading folklore concerning self-care and health. As intelligent people we want to do what is best, but the folklore interferes. Let's look at some of our most common twentieth century fables in the light of facts.

STRESS

Stress is being overstressed. Not only can we tolerate difficulties in our daily living, we need them. The kind of stress that kills occurred far more frequently when our ancestors lived in caves with only a stick to protect them from tigers. They lived through it and learned how to turn the tiger into a coat in the process, thus bettering themselves in every way. So can we.

Severe mental stress can lead to a personality breakdown, it's true; but it can also lead to the path of an Einstein or a Fermi—all the great men and women of yesterday and today.

Nor is mental stress really that unnerving. For most of us, it can be the spur that forces us to solve personal problems with satisfaction and joy, rather than merely hoping they will be solved by somebody else.

The Greek philosophers observed years ago that there should be "moderation in all things," and moderation is our defense against stress. When too much stress comes our way in one direction, we should look for tasks to do in another direction. This was what Freud meant when he talked of sublimation. If one task or one situation overwhelms you with tension, walk out on it. Go out and take a good walk, swim, play a game of tennis. Some physical outlet to blow off steam. Then come back fresh and unwound. The trouble may still be waiting for you—or it may have gone away during your absence, as it so often surprisingly does.

Stress and the drives of life are inseparable. The way to win the battle with stress is by preparation, onslaught, and renewal to attack again; not by retiring to a life in a cocoon of cotton candy and inactivity. Taking up a hobby, or a specialized study that interests us, will give us another outlet in which to put our stress to work, rather than being overwhelmed by it.

FATIGUE

In the healthy person physical fatigue is cured by rest. If rest does not remove such fatigue, your health is suspect and a thorough examination by your physician is in order.

Mental fatigue responds to a change of mental scenery. No one has ever demonstrated this better than Sir Isaac Newton. He was completely stumped on a mathematics problem, and decided to go for a walk in his garden. There, as all of us know, he saw the apple fall and realized the existence of gravity—a momentous discovery made by a mentally-fatigued brain.

We don't always need the garden walk to change our mental scenery, but we do need the willingness to change our train of thoughts to new subjects.

WHAT ABOUT ALCOHOL?

There are other bits of misinformation and half-information that worry us in our search for a long, happy life. They worry us because we hear all sorts of statements about what we should and shouldn't do to reach our goal of a hundred happy years.

Certainly high on most lists of worries is the question of alcohol. Let us approach it from this point of view:

There are three places in the world today where an active life lasting well past a century is a frequent experience. Blatten, Switzerland; Hunza in the Himalayas; and the Thar, the desert of India and West Pakistan. Although we know very little of the people of the Thar, the Swiss and the Hunzing as both use alcoholic beverages—not to wild excess, but with both regularity and enjoyment.

Another fact of interest on this topic is found in France. Although the average French citizen's diet is quite high in fat, the French have less disease of the heart and arteries than do other people with such large quantities of fat in their diet. It may be that they are protected by the wine they drink —either by the wine itself, or because many of their calories come from the wine, and the over-all proportion of fat they eat is somewhat less than it seems when only solid food is taken into account.

Let us be fair. Wine, and other alcoholic beverages are of use to many. The dangers of alcoholism cannot be ignored, but fortunately they are the problem of a few. Wine has been called the milk of the elderly, and it has been known to help a number of digestive problems. It has even been used, in some cases, as a treatment for alcoholism. Again, we must repeat our Golden Rule—Moderation.

CIGARETTES AND TOBACCO

They are today's best-publicized health problems, and we all want an answer. Some people say they know the answer: cigarettes cause cancer of the lung, and that is that.

Others point out that the heaviest smokers of cigarettes known are South Africans of European descent, and these people have a subnormally low frequency of lung cancer. Cigarette manufacturers' employees, who have been studied for years, and who smoke heavily, also have a lower incidence of lung cancer than might be expected.

The answer is plain: no one knows the answer today; so, again, the best advice is—Moderation.

There are, however, some diseases where the arteries of the body can be put into a spasm readily, and smoking will make these matters worse. In such cases, tobacco must be avoided. That is the only definite medical information we have about tobacco.

VITAMINS

Commercial vitamins are a highly publicized discovery of the twentieth century. What they really amount to are very small amounts of chemicals that the body needs to properly use foods.

For most of us, making a daily habit of some good vitamin preparation is necessary. Too often we eat meals that have been cooked too long, or prepared with more attention to appearance than to nutrition. A pre-meal cocktail also may be doing its part in washing out the vitamins in our foods.

The person who eats all of his meals in a home environment with good preparation and balance does not usually need these supplements. Unfortunately, most of us eat few of our meals under such ideal circumstances and therefore, for most of us, a good vitamin supplement is necessary.

Chapter Seventeen

THE WISH TO DESTROY OURSELVES—
HOW TO DETECT AND AVOID IT

Many of us still regard death with a casual fatalism that might bring envy to many an Eastern mind. Although the Hindu confidently expects a long life in which to continue his study of self, too many of us Westerners over 35 act "as if there were no tomorrow," and take chances and inflict punishments on our own bodies that appall our doctors. Simply changing this mental attitude can go far toward improving our chances of reaching one hundred.

SUICIDE

Suicide accounts for about seven per cent of adult deaths in the United States each year. Suicide is not a disease, but many suicides are preventable.

The first step in its prevention is simply to know something about its causes. Emotional disorders, particularly depressions, are largely responsible for self-destruction. By depression, physicians mean a deep-seated feeling of unworthiness and despair. Such a condition can arise quite suddenly "out of nowhere," and be just as fatal as another depression that has lasted for years. Its recognition is the key to treatment.

"Why go on living when things are all wrong?"—that is the question the suicide cannot correctly answer. Somehow the ordinary satisfactions of life and its great joys are completely hidden—only the bad can be seen. When this happens the individual needs help—wise and trained assistance. The psychiatrist, or physician, the priest, rabbi or minister —these are the people to go to for guidance. They are the ones able to restore our ability to see *all* of life instead of maintaining the one-sided view that has led to thoughts of leaving it.

CAR ACCIDENTS—THEY CAN BE PREVENTED

Emotional hygiene through definite and reasonable mental goals is the way back from thoughts of self-destruction. Not only from the direct suicide that some consciously plan, but accidental deaths that needlessly take so many other lives.

As one vital example, take safety belts. Their acceptance —or rejection—is entirely a matter of emotional adjustment.

In a nation of 60 million cars, our exposure to driving hazards is continuous. The fact of thirty-eight thousand deaths per year—now totaling one and a half million deaths in the United States since 1900—is a shocking figure. We have lost in war far less lives than this.

The number of deaths prevented by seat belts every year is an equally impressive figure. In 1961 the National Safety Council estimated that about 5000 lives had been saved by these devices. And yet they are worn by only a fraction of a per cent of all drivers!

In addition, life may be rather hard to live through by a person with only half a face—or one who is chained to a wheelchair. One and a half million people are injured each year in auto accidents.

Wearing safety belts will not only lessen the numbers injured—but, far more important, those who are injured will have far less permanent disfigurement and damage. Talk to a few people who have been smashed up—you'll never find one who doesn't wish he had worn a seat belt. Let's start our own war on the misuse of the car—if only to save our lives.

ALCOHOL AND ACCIDENTS

Not all accidents occur in cars, nor will the seat belt cure all automobile deaths. Alcohol will put a fog on the road that no one should try to drive through. At two drinks most people have enough alcohol in their blood to give a recording of 0.1%. And such a blood alcohol level of 0.1% constitutes *Prima Facia* evidence of drunken driving in many states.

With alcohol in the blood, as many as four distinct changes take place in the personality. Alcohol is an anesthetic, not a stimulant, and it acts the same as any other anesthetic. First, drowsiness; second, excitement; third, sleep; fourth, death. These are also the four levels of anesthesia.

We drink for the effects of the first and second stages; but we can slip past these into the fourth far too easily as we sit behind our steering wheels. Vision becomes blurred, and we see a smaller and smaller view on either side. Judgment of distances and of situations is impaired. Reaction time—the mind to muscle action route—is slowed up. If you drink, driving and killing are not heroic—and it's not the fault of someone else—it's your fault.

A LITTLE CARE—A LONG LIFE

There are lots of other gay and popular ways of doing yourself in. Scuba diving, water skiing, small planes—all of these have been found to be fatal if mishandled. Something similar to Knute Rockne's saying is appropriate here: "It's not what you're doing, but how much you know about it that makes the game."

The wise and cautious person first learns the equipment, its limitations, and, above all, his own limitations.

In many of our occupations and recreations there are legal requirements for a license, and these should be passed with honesty if you have any real regard for your own life and limb. In most other areas of recreation there are well qualified experts willing to show you the mastery of whatever art you wish to know. Use them.

Hunting is an outdoor, any-weather, rugged, simple sport, yet many lose their lives each year by disregarding its fundamental rules. A lack of such wisdom frequently causes someone to be fatally shot by a stranger or friend with more speed than sense. Others put their own guns to the task of finishing their lives—not on purpose, but out of sheer carelessness. And, of course, the prime killer of your time—the heart attack—walks the woods these days and claims many a weekend athlete.

BEWARE THE WEEKEND STRAIN

Other occasional activities can also have unfortunate and unexpected results, if we are not prepared.

Winter time, with its snow shoveling and car pushing activities, gives us all a certain amount of scare copy in the news. The best guide line for your ability to shovel snow was that provided by the New York State Medical Journal about a year ago.

This article stated that no one who did not walk at least one continuous mile every day of his life should attempt to shovel snow.

I would like to add the advice given earlier on fatigue. Many of us know that the best way to do a mental job is all at once—to see it through. Not so with physical activities; when you become tired—quit. Go back and finish the job later, rather than push on, heedlessly, never to finish.

Pushing a car is another example. Certainly only those in a real condition of fitness should try. Even if you are in good shape, don't try to push any car too hard; wait for a truck, or a team—let the expert have his livelihood too. Your physician would much rather see you for your regular health audit in the spring.

WEATHER AND YOUR HEART

Winter is the time of the greatest number of heart attacks in the north, because the weather itself is a strain.

In the south the heat and humidity cause a greater strain in the summer—and that is when their physicians record the greatest number of heart attacks. Therefore, avoid strenuous activity in extremes of weather—either cold or hot.

This life is yours; maintain it correctly, and no one will know greater joy. Slip for a moment, and you may have to substitute a long time of grief in overfull repayment of a brief error.

The motto of IBM is still good—THINK.

Chapter Eighteen

HOW TO TAKE CARE OF YOUR BACK

Doing things the wrong way seems to come naturally to most of us. We have been given bad examples from our childhood days. Also, we are too weak, too lacking in muscular power to think of doing things the right way.

Nowhere is this more true than in the use we make of our backs. Many of us know how to use our backs correctly; yet we can't be bothered to utilize this knowledge when we pick up or carry something. There may even be group ridicule for anyone who decides to use his back correctly.

A UNIVERSAL PROBLEM

These problems of the correct use of the back are not confined to the occasional individual who does heavy manual labor: they are common to all of us.

The housewife, standing at a sink, or picking up her baby, exposes her back to as many hazards as does the construction laborer. She may even incur a greater danger, for she has less to help her in the way of machinery.

Also, her husband, with his enforced hobbies of storm window fitting and lawn care, may really know less about taking care of his back than any foreman would tolerate in his workers.

The commonest causes of financial loss to employers and

insurance companies are back problems, all of which are preventable—and such prevention is of far more importance to you, who might suffer the pain and disability, than it is to your employer or insuror. Let's take care of *every* part of the body in our daily living.

THE ONE BASIC RULE

Lift with your knees, not with your back. Everyone of us has heard this statement. It is true! It is true *all* the time! When you stoop over to lift with your back it is at once a confession of weakness and of ignorance. Let's take a look at the wrong, and right, ways to do our lifting:

THE WRONG WAY

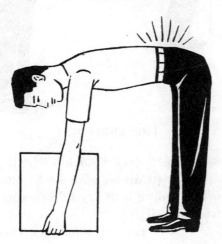

This is the way everybody wants to do it. This gives us diseases for which no "shot" or immune vaccine has been, or ever will be, developed.

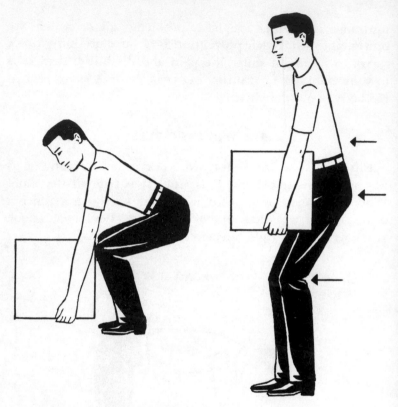

THE RIGHT WAY

It's really so simple! Back straight. BEND at the knees. You never place the strain on your back—the legs take all the weight for you. Doing it this right way, you can lift twice the weight, twice as easily.

Incidentally, a good part of your back care has already begun with the specific exercise program outlined. The proper tricks of walking are just as important as the exercises themselves if you are really to put this program of back care into action. Your increased flexibility and strength will make it easy for you to lift, carry, move the objects that fate puts in your path daily.

THE RIGHT WAY TO LIFT A WEIGHT OVER YOUR HEAD

A. Stick out your hands. Bend at the knees. Take hold.

B. One leg back—straight as you push up with your arms.

C. Legs in line, far enough apart for balance. Arms straighten up—over head.

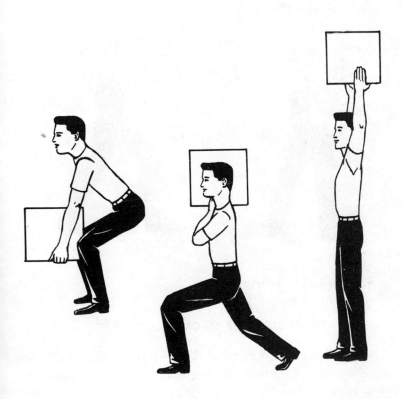

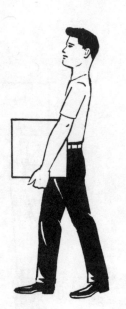 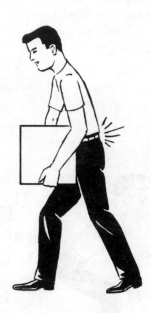

THE RIGHT WAY TO CARRY A WEIGHT

When you carry, keep your back straight, and walk the same way you do when not loaded down. This not only spares your back, but lets you carry a heavy load a longer distance before you tire.

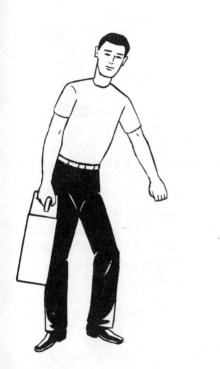
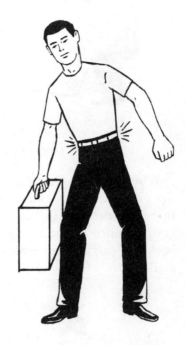

IF THE LOAD HAS A HANDLE

Some of our problems of lifting and carrying come equipped with handles. Tilt your body in a straight line to the side; don't bend in the middle to dodge the load.

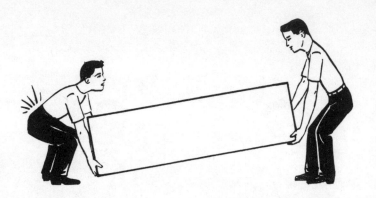

HOW TWO PEOPLE SHOULD NOT LIFT

When two people pick up something, they both must lift the right way. The man on the right has lifted so quickly that the man on the left, although in proper position, is getting more of the weight and strain of the load than his back can carry. The result—Pain! Lift together—slowly and easily.

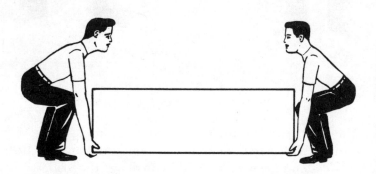

THE CORRECT SHOULDER CARRY

When carrying something on your shoulder don't always use the same side of your body. If you do you will get lopsided—as the hod carriers did in years gone by.

OTHER WEIGHTS

A case of wine brings no joy if the back, and not the knees, is bent to carry it.

The pail may be empty or full; the back can be hurt by the lightest of loads if the load is carried wrong.

IN SUMMARY

Your back doesn't need to be greased every 1000 miles, but it can be good for a lifetime, when properly used.

Chapter Nineteen

OH BELOVED—AND BENEFICIAL—SLEEP

How much sleep do we need for vibrant health? This question has intrigued mankind through the ages. But only recently has research given us most of the answers we need. Some of them will certainly startle you.

WHAT LACK OF SLEEP DOES TO US

Sometimes the newspapers seem to confound our ordinary impressions about the necessity of sleep with reports of some elderly person who has gone without sleep for most of his or her adult life. These people are the geniuses—the rare exceptions that we can admire, but should not imitate.

Sleep is a necessity of life, not a luxury. Too little sleep can result in the symptoms of a starvation even more dramatic than the symptoms caused by fasting from food. If sleeplessness is attempted for any prolonged period, our bodies will fail in one way or another.

Ten days of fasting from food has been tolerated—well tolerated—by numbers of people. But ten days without sleep does not mean ten days of moderate discomfort, such as might be expected from a fast of this length. During these ten days the most mentally alert become confused, see imaginary objects, actually act insane. Even after these experimenters have had rest, it may be weeks before all their mental processes are restored to normal.

WILL CAT NAPS DO?

Stories of short sleeping hours are well known in the cases of Churchill, Edison and Napoleon. Not so well known is the fact that daytime naps were part of the schedules of all these men, and a twenty-four hour record would usually show that they spent six to eight hours at rest.

Most of us find it more convenient to do all our sleeping at once, rather than in various segments throughout the day. However way we choose, we all must take a minimum amount of rest each day if we are to maintain our health.

SLEEP AND LONGEVITY

The benefits of sleep are dramatically illustrated in the story of the humming bird. At the rate this tiny creature burns up energy when awake, it could only live two or three hours without food. However, during sleep, the humming bird's energy requirements are diminished to a point where it can sleep through the entire night without danger of starvation. When the humming bird sleeps, it enters a state of sleep far deeper than do humans. It can slow its energy requirements down greatly by nearly freezing during the night.

This method of survival has been of interest to many scientists, particularly those interested in longevity. Russian

experimenters in the early fifties attempted to see what
effect prolonged sleep could have on longevity.

They obtained a fifteen year old dog, very near the end of
its natural life span. Not only was it old, it showed signs of
great age—falling hair, poor appetite, listless behavior.

Through sedatives, and perhaps also the use of cold, this
animal was put to sleep for ninety days—and gained a new
lease on life. It regained the vigor and hair of its middle
years, and lived another six and one-half years. Death, when
it came, was not from natural causes, but occurred during
a fight with a chimpanzee.

ONE HUNDRED EIGHTY-ONE YEARS OLD!

This was a startling experiment, and its true meaning can
be best realized by translating it into human terms. A dog,
at fifteen years, is as old, in many ways, as a human at one
hundred and twenty-five. Each—dog and man—have at that
time lived to five times the age it took for their skeletons to
mature. This is the length of time, from many scientific
viewpoints, in which each is supposed to have lived his full
life span.

Adding the six and one-half years to the dog's life, then,
would be equal to adding better than fifty-six years to a
man's life—a grand total of one hundred eighty-one years!

The only major drawback would be to find the old man
who can be given this artificial sleep for about twenty-one
years—for that would be the right proportion to the dog's
ninety days.

How much a long sleep in the cold is worth may have
also been demonstrated by the three groups known to have
extremely long life spans in the world today. Both the Swiss
and the Hunzingas live in mountainous territories where

cold nights and a lack of heat are a regular part of their life.

The other long-lived group may at first seem an enigma: the people who live in the Indian desert. However, deserts, though known for their great heat at mid-day, are barren of most plant life because of their cold at night. So the Rajasthani and other inhabitants of the desert also have a cold sleep every night.

This cold may be one of the sources of their longevity; or, of course, it may not. More work has to be done on the whole subject before more than speculation can be offered.

HOW MUCH SLEEP DO YOU NEED?

We were all taught in school that eight hours sleep was considered the right and proper amount. It is a good average figure, but cannot be stated with absolute certainty to apply to each and every one of us at all times.

Neither can we point to various individuals who are getting along on less than eight hours and state with certainty that they are doing what is best—even for themselves. It is not hard to find numbers of doctors who feel strongly that too little sleep is frequently associated with a shortened life span.

Nor, again, can we prove that great amounts of sleep lead to a much improved length of life—although there is that impression in the minds of many.

Seven to nine hours' sleep is the amount of rest that most people need to feel refreshed and alert day after day. All of us have days when less than this is sufficient, and most of us also have days when quite a bit more would seem desirable.

INSOMNIA, AND WHAT TO DO ABOUT IT

The problem of both sleep and its enemy, insomnia, will become far less troublesome when you are in good physical condition. Keeping your body in tune during the day will aid it to serve you better through all the twenty-four hours.

Sleeplessness is regarded with more concern than is usually justified. An occasional inability to fall into deep sleep is common with nearly everyone. Resting quietly in bed at such times can give us the minimum of relaxation and renewal we need for the next day.

However, if such insomnia persists, it deserves to be called a habit rather than a disease. This pattern, frequent in older persons, can be bothersome for all concerned. Chronic sleeplessness at night can result in a foggy, half-awake day, sure to be followed by another poor night.

This vicious circle can be broken by making sure wakefulness is assured during the day. Coffee and tea both will wake up even the drowsiest; use them in adequate amounts for breakfast and the mid-day meal. Add some definite, purposeful activity during the day-time hours. Prepare for a night's sleep by filling the day with action.

Of course, even a wide-awake day will not guarantee everyone a full night's sleep. Some individuals demand more than ordinary activity to enjoy complete rest. A full program of physical fitness is the only answer for 99% of their problems. Their bodies need heavy muscular exertion for good physical and mental health.

If every bit of this advice has been tried, and success still eludes you, then it is time to seek medical help. There are diseases that can keep us from sleep, and the longer they are given the opportunity to exhaust us, the more seriously they will harm our health.

Chapter Twenty

IS IT TRUE WHAT THEY SAY ABOUT WALKING?

When President John F. Kennedy made his famous statement about fifty-mile hikes he little realized that he would get the nation on its feet once more—in more ways than one. Newspapers all over the country were deluged with reports about college men hiking fifty miles, Marines doing the fifty-mile stint and persons in all walks of life (to make a bad pun) began to walk. But no one really stopped to think about the real benefits of walking. Certainly a business man who had been "chained" behind his desk could not and should not go in for long extended walks or hikes. But there is so much to be said about walking and its beneficial effects on the human body that I would like to set forth the following:

Can walking help you grow slender (and stay slender) the rest of your life without dieting?

Can walking help you reduce your blood cholesterol and your blood pressure without dieting?

Can walking possibly help you reduce your chance of stroke or heart attack?

Yes, it probably can! And there is a good chance that it will . . . IF . . . if you are willing to walk enough!

Beyond this one inescapable fact there are no tricks . . . no special diets . . . no drugs . . . no counting calories!

Very well then, you say: "How much walking must I do?" You may have heard it said that you must walk 36 miles to lose one pound of fat. And, being accustomed to weighing the pros and cons of a proposition, you are inclined to ask: "Is it worth it?"

FIRST, AS TO YOUR WEIGHT . . .

Look at it this way. Would you be willing to walk a mile a day . . . requiring some 15 minutes of your time if you walk briskly . . . to lose nearly a pound a month . . . 10 pounds in a year?

Would you be willing to walk half an hour a day briskly (15 minutes to and from your office, for example) in order to lose 20 pounds in 12 months?

Can you afford to take the time to walk 5 miles a day, all at one time or half in the morning and half in the evening, in order to lose a pound a week, 4 pounds in a month? Or perhaps you should ask yourself, can I afford NOT to?

Why? Because losing weight, getting down to fighting trim, is just one benefit of walking an hour or so a day. Studies indicate an hour or so of exercise a day can help you reduce your blood cholesterol, help you reduce your blood pressure, and help you reduce your risk of a stroke or heart attack.

ON STAVING OFF THE INEVITABLE . . .

Perhaps you have heard it said that exercise after 40 is unnecessary and, in fact, may be dangerous. Each winter the newspapers report the deaths of a number of men from heart attacks while shoveling snow. And, by implication, it is the snow-shoveling that gets the blame. Now it is true that sudden strenuous exercise can be harmful if you are not in reasonably good condition. But completely overlooked is the fact that other men had heart attacks the day before any particular snowstorm, and the day after; and that they occur every day in Southern California where it rarely snows. But the newspapers never report that Mr. X died of a heart attack "from NOT shoveling snow." Likely as not he was watching television!

What guarantee, you may ask, is there that our not-so-mythical Mr. X if he had exercised regularly would have lived longer? Admittedly, none. Obviously, he could have had the misfortune to step in front of the wrong automobile, slip on a wet step, or . . . perhaps . . . be shot by a jealous husband (which, at 80, is reputed to be not a bad way to go). But it is more than mere conjecture that, even if he were predisposed to cardiac disease, he might have staved off the inevitable, perhaps for many years, by regular daily exercise.

WHAT ABOUT THE TIME?

Now you may be thinking, what you say may be fine but I simply do not have the time to fit a regular program of exercise into my schedule . . . certainly not an hour's walk a day. Fair enough . . . but first let's get this much straight! If you happen to be the type who works up to 16 hours a day, whether from devotion to duty or because you feel you are indispensable, perhaps the best we can say is, "Good luck!" But, if you want to improve your chances of living longer . . . and really living, not just existing . . . you must find the time to keep fit.

Sure, it is a problem, a tough one! But your job as an executive (the thing that has counted most in your ability to put yourself where you are) has required an unusual flair for solving problems. Surely . . . when your future, your very life depends upon it . . . you can find some way to solve this problem of enough time.

Perhaps, before you tackle this time problem, you look for an alternative. You say to yourself . . . "What about this walking to reduce, isn't there some quicker way to lose weight?"

There are several! At intervals you can, for example, abstain completely from eating for several days (in a hospital under a doctor's supervision) . . . and there are crash diets and weight-reducing pills (also requiring medical supervision). But more important, few people have the will-power to adhere to a strict dietary regimen and, what is more, even if you have the will-power, for an executive, it often isn't very practical. The luncheon conferences, the cocktail parties, the entertaining of business associates, would seem to make exercise rather than diet the better method for you.

In fact, dieting without exercise, may be unwise. Continual hunger and dissatisfaction with the limitations imposed by a diet do nothing to condition the heart and lead to frustration. A fashion-model agency director has put it this way: "When a woman goes on a diet, it is not her bones but her nerves that stick out first!"

WHAT ABOUT THE FACTS?

Perhaps it is time to take a look at the facts behind our assurances that this walking will pay off.

First, you, your body economy, can be considered as a business. You put in a certain amount of raw material—food . . . and have (usually) a fairly constant output in terms of physical and mental activity. And in the process you accumulate a reserve . . . all too frequently too much of a reserve . . . of fat.

Your "reserve"may look a little trimmer than the next fellow's (thanks to your tailor) but 20 or 30 pounds of excess fat are 20 or 30 pounds too much . . . as life insurance mortality tables prove so brutally.

Since one pound of body fat is the fairly precise equivalent of 3500 calories, if you are 30 pounds over your ideal weight (approximately what you weighed at 25) you have a "reserve" of about 100,000 calories to burn off just to get back to your most efficient level of doing business.

As pointed out earlier, you can lose a pound a week (and in some 30 weeks burn up your 100,000 calories "reserve") if you will walk 5 miles a day every day.

BUT WHAT ABOUT YOUR APPETITE?

Another question probably occurs to you. If I walk 5 miles a day won't this additional exercise (and it must be in addition to however much walking you do now) increase my appetite and defeat my purpose?

No . . . *it will not! The fact is* (for people like yourself who are anchored at a desk most of the day) *increased exercise does not increase appetite in proportion!*

WEIGHT CONTROL ONLY THE BEGINNING!

Weight control is essential but regular exercise has other vital benefits. Combined they can greatly increase your vigor and efficiency . . . help you to a far longer and more enjoyable "prime of life."

First, there are the immediate physical effects of regular daily walks on the circulation. Good muscle tone in the arms and particularly in the legs, resulting from hourly walks, maintains an improved circulation of blood in the veins. Since the veins have valves, which when in good condition prevent the blood from going the wrong way, the compression of the veins by the skeletal muscles during walking helps to pump the blood back to the heart. Soft, unused muscles do not do this job as well, and they also make clogging in the veins more likely . . . as when one sits for a long time or when an operation or an illness keeps one inactive. (That is why it is best, for example, on long trips by train or plane or car to get up or out and walk a bit at intervals to combat this tendency.) Thrombosis (clogging) in the leg veins can have serious consequences when part of a clot breaks off and blocks an important blood vessel in one's lung.

Vigorous daily walks also improve the tone of the diaphragm, which results in its better function as the piston of a pump, not only for bringing oxygen to the lungs with removal of carbon dioxide, but also for the suction of blood into the heart.

Another part of the circulatory apparatus helped by regular long walks is that of the smallest blood vessels . . . the arterioles, the capillaries and the venules . . . which are thus rendered more active in their function. The peripheral vessels of the hands, the feet and the ears react beneficially with

less likelihood of sluggishness and slackening of the blood
flow. Although the heart is the main agent in maintaining
circulation, the aid it receives from these other structures is
considerable and may on occasion mean the difference between good health and physical unfitness.

There are other beneficial effects of a long daily walk.
Digestion and bowel function are improved; vigorous walks
often render laxative medicine quite unnecessary. And a long
brisk walk in the evening may help more to induce sleep than
any medicine.

An intense mental worker needs exercise to keep his mind
clear. Mental concentration should be alternated with
exercise.

One of the most important of all benefits, especially for
an executive, is the effect of regular daily exercise on the
nervous system. It has been said that a 5 mile walk will do
more good to a worried or unhappy but healthy man than
all the medicine and psychology in the world. Nervous stress
and strain can be counteracted and even prevented by regular
vigorous daily walks.

EXERCISE, CHOLESTEROL AND MENTAL ALERTNESS

Several recent studies indicate the role that regular daily
exercise can play in lowering blood cholesterol and the role
that cholesterol plays in mental altertness.

The first is a report, mentioned by Alvarez, of six months'
study of 30 men who started with an average blood cholesterol level of 251 miligrams. They took each day an hour of
exercise, and wound up with an average blood cholesterol
level of 195 miligrams. A control group of 30 men who ate
a similar diet, but did not exercise, had no change in their
blood cholesterol.

The second is a report of 42 middle-aged white-collar workers whose average cholesterol levels were far above normal. After a year of an hour's exercise 5 days a week the average drop in the group was from 261 to 195, with individuals going from nearly 300 to around 150. The changes were in direct proportion to attendance. It becomes obvious that physical fitness is much more than strength such as is found in laborers. It is the building up of endurance, lung power and muscle tissue.

The third report is by investigators at the University of Chicago Clinics who found that men over 45 with high blood cholesterol are less alert than men with low cholesterol. Eleven psychological tests were used to measure the two groups' reasoning ability, problem solving, reaction time, and time sense. This seems related to the fact that hardening of the arteries affects the blood vessels of the brain and thus interferes with the brain cells' functioning.

THE ONLY WAY TO EXERCISE A BLOOD VESSEL

Your blood vessels are lined with smooth muscle fibers and, if these smooth muscles do not get exercise, they atrophy just like any other part of the body. But the only way you can exercise a blood vessel is to put a demand on the blood stream for oxygen. You do physical exercise and your muscular tissues use up oxygen. Your heart has to beat faster to pump along a new supply of oxygen-carrying blood to meet the demand. As your heart increases its pumping action it pushes more blood through your system; and the blood vessels expand to allow this more profuse circulation. Later they contract. And this expansion and contraction is exercise!

EFFECT OF EXERCISE ON BLOOD PRESSURE

An hour's daily walk not only exercises your blood vessels, this long-continued contracting of the muscles increases the flow of blood in the body and its return to the heart. The heart responds with a greater contracting force calling forth better circulation within the heart itself and the opening of more blood vessels. The increased number of channels for blood to flow through results in less resistance to flow, and as a result, a reduction in blood pressure.

Even men in middle-age who have not exercised regularly in many years can achieve a marked reduction in blood pressure through a carefully-graduated increase in their daily walks. Hearts which, like President Eisenhower's, have suffered blockage of an artery apparently can be stimulated by such carefully-graduated exercise to sprout new artery branches.

For some time now it has been known that when a coronary artery that feeds blood to the heart muscle is narrowed or even blocked, the heart usually provides its own system of repairs. It does this through growth of arteries near the danger area and through the sprouting of new artery branches. These collateral blood vessels take over the job of supplying the heart muscle with blood. How to encourage this growth of collateral blood vessels has been an important question. Now a slow, graduated increase in daily exercise from merely walking around the hospital room to walking around the block and eventually to walking from 2 to 5 miles a day is growing in favor.

WHAT ABOUT HARDENING OF THE ARTERIES?

Regular daily exercise is apparently helpful in preventing hardening of the arteries. A study of 500 prominent U.S. athletes who still exercise in middle age shows that they have little or no sign of artery disease compared with other men their same ages.

The Valley Forge Heart Institute conducted another study of participants from 17 to 67 years old in two marathon races. Particular attention was paid to impacts on the cardiovascular system. Using the very latest testing methods and instrumentation, the runners were examined before and after the races with a special view to the possible effects of "wear and tear" in relation to the so-called degenerative diseases. In runners over the age 40 there were no signs whatever of the onset of atherosclerosis, the form of hardening of the arteries so common among men above 40 who are not physically active. It was clear that strenuous physical activity over prolonged years, far from hastening the degenerative diseases associated with aging, actually prevents and inhibits these symptoms.

THE ANTI-OLD-AGE "ANTIBIOTIC" . . .

Such studies show why it is important to remember that nothing remains static that is biological. If you do not use a part of the body, it atrophies. As Dr. Ernst Jokl has remarked: "We have discovered an age-inhibiting factor so important in forestalling the effects of old age that it might be termed the anti-old-age antibiotic. This anti-age antibiotic is free. It is regular daily exercise."

So today, after some 2,000 years, a long series of medical

studies here and abroad is verifying that Hippocrates was right. Regular exercise, especially walking, is man's best "medicine."

Hippocrates mentions walking 40 times in one chapter on the digestive diseases. He prescribes brisk walks, short walks, early morning walks, after-dinner walks, night walks. Early morning walks were for emotional disturbances. Brisk walks were to reduce weight and keep one's figure trim.

Walking was described by the Greek writer, Pliny the Elder, as one of the "Medicines of the Will" . . . and it still is. For you have to have will-power enough to take it (walking) every day.

How is it that Hippocrates' advice was so long ignored? After the luxury and the soft-living of the golden days of Greece and Rome, at least for some segments of those civilizations, the world fell on terrible times. Even two or three generations ago, our ancestors took a lot of exercise routinely in their lives. They thought little of walking 5 or 10 miles, or of cycling 25, or of working hard on the farm all day, or of going into the woods and working for hours cutting down trees. That was more or less the routine life, and all of a sudden, in one generation, has come this rather abrupt change. Today we ride instead of walk . . . gadgets have taken over where muscles were always used.

That so many, many generations who worked so much harder had so much shorter a life expectancy than the one we can anticipate is another matter. Exercise cannot compensate for poor nutrition, poor sanitation, and an utter lack of preventive medicine.

NOW TO SUM UP:

Walking is a special kind of experience . . . long walks! Once you have formed the habit, you'll understand as no one else's words can tell you.

But remember, in order for your walks to be effective as a therapeutic agent, to strengthen your nerve-muscle tone and stimulate your cardio-respiratory system, you must carry them out with regularity . . . and if you haven't exercised for many years regularly, your muscles need a gradual awakening to the demand you will put upon them.

How can you know how much exercise is too much? You have a built-in mechanism that is a reliable indicator, one which automatically adjusts itself to your increasing capacities. This is what is known as your "Recovery Rate."

Even for a conditioned athlete, pulse and respiration rate will rise with increased activity, but return to normal quickly at rest.

Regardless of your physical state at any given time, you should exercise only enough to permit your heart and breathing to return to normal quickly after you stop. So, remember, exercising has been too strenuous if:

— your heart refuses to stop pounding 10 minutes after exercising . . .
— your breathing is still uncomfortable 10 minutes after exercising . . .
— you are still shaky for more than 30 minutes after exercising . . .
— you cannot sleep well the night after exercising . . .
— you carry fatigue (not muscle soreness) into the next day . . .

If any of these stages persist, it is a sign that you should take it easier for awhile.

After a week or two of walking one to three miles at a slow pace, you should be ready to walk 3 to 5 miles at a brisk pace with little difficulty. In 6 to 8 weeks the pace should be increased so that it will take approximately an hour to walk 3½ miles.

A leisurely pace is around 3 miles per hour. A brisk walk usually averages 3½ miles per hour.

If walking is continued for 3 months, you should then be able to walk 4 miles in an hour on alternate days, and 3 miles per hour the others. This break in routine is good mental relaxation as well as good training procedure.

In order to increase your work-out, you need only to walk up a grade or hill. It has been shown that it is easier to increase work with increasing the incline than to increase the pace; for above 4 miles per hour most individuals must jog or run.

By timing the distance you walk or by counting the number of steps you take per minute, you can easily establish your approximate pace. You may remember, too, that military pace is usually 120 steps to the minute . . . and this pace amounts to, roughly, 3½ miles to the hour.

* * * * *

Is it true what they say about walking? The poets seem never to have forgotten the human situation . . . in their reflections upon the nature of things. Long ago, for example, Dryden observed: "The wise for cure on exercise depend." And our own Robert Frost (when 87) smilingly remarked: "I have walked many miles with my dog. It has done me a lot of good. I hope it has my dog."

Our last suggestion. When you walk, walk as if your life depended upon it . . . for it does!

* * * * *

REFERENCES

1. Bortz, E. L., Mechanisms of Aging, *J. of the American Geriatrics Society*, 7:825, (1959).
2. Brouha, L., Physiology of Training, Including Age and Sex Differences, *J. of Sports Medicine and Physical Fitness*, 2:3, (1962).
3. *Exercise and Fitness*, Chicago, The Athletic Institute, (1960).
4. Johnson, T. F. et al., The Influence of Exercise on Serum Cholesterol, Phospholipids, and Electrophoretic Serum Protein Patterns in College Swimmers. *Proceedings Federation of American Societies for Experimental Biology*, 18:77, (1959).
5. Johnson, W. R., editor, *Science and Medicine of Exercise and Sports*, Harper and Brothers, New York, (1960).
6. Karvonen, M. J., *Ergonomics*, 2:207, (1959).
7. Mayer, J. et al., Relation between caloric intake, body weight and physical work, *American Journal of Clinical Nutrition*, 4:169, (1956).
8. Michael, E. D., Stress Adaptation Through Exercise, *Research Quarterly*, 28:50, (1957).
9. Morris, J. N. et al., Coronary Heart Disease and Physical Activity of Work, *Lancet*, 265:1053, (1953).
10. Rook, A., An Investigation into the Longevity of Cambridge Sportsmen, *British Medical Journal*, 1:773, (1954).

Chapter Twenty-One

WHAT'S HOLDING YOU BACK?

If there was a single magic pill or "shot" that would immediately and automatically assure you of a long, vigorous life, you would want to purchase it, no matter what its cost. You would pay any sum of money to live longer.

At the turn of the century, when advertising was in its infancy, and less sophistication and education were common, this promise of "long life in a bottle" was offered by hundreds of promoters. In those days, although the product wouldn't work, the promise did. People would rush out and buy snake root, swamp grass, liver bile—or any other nauseating mixture the medicine man had compounded. They would accept any promise to live longer.

EXCUSES THAT HELP US DIG OUR OWN GRAVE

But today we "know better"—we laugh at the promise of a long, healthy, vigorous life. We protect our own flabbiness and potential disaster with standard excuses like these:

One: "Whenever I feel like exercising I lie down until the feeling goes away."

Two: "I find my exercise in acting as pallbearer for my friends who exercise."

Three: "I keep fit by winding my watch—but I may get a self-winding model to spare my muscles."

Four: "I only exercise discretion."

Five: "It cost a lot for me to get into this shape, I have to keep it now as an investment."

Feeble excuses which only hide our own inner knowledge that we are shortening our lives, deliberately and inevitably.

DON'T HIDE BEHIND A WOMAN'S SKIRTS

"Women live longer than men in any case, so what chance do we guys have?"—another common excuse.

Women *do* outlive men in the United States, and in much of the Western world. But men outlive women in Finland and in New Zealand. And all these statistics are only the *current*, twentieth-century figures on mortality.

There is no such thing as a biological superiority of females over males. Whatever hereditary differences there are between men and women do not lengthen or shorten life. It is what you do with your body, not what kind of body you are given, that counts in the long run!

CAN YOU "OVER DO" THIS PROGRAM?

There is also the common fear of "overdoing" a fitness program—of "straining something"—that worries many. This can be dispelled with these facts:

1) No one has ever been able to prove the occurrence of a heart attack in an athlete—in condition—*at any age.* (Ath-

letes out of condition are in the same boat with the rest of us, of course.)

2) In Finland it has been shown, many times, that those who ski live several years longer than those who do not.

3) Physical training not only makes us feel better but is *the only way* the body chemistry can be kept in good condition.

SO LITTLE TIME—SUCH WONDERFUL RESULTS!

"I don't have time"—there's the pathetic final excuse! Unfortunately it's just not true. We always have a few moments of time to add quite a few more years to our lives.

All you need is three half-hours each week. If this amount of time could not have been found by most of us a few years ago, nobody would have purchased a television set.

The question is, then, where shall we allot the time for this physical activity? As far as our bodies are concerned, it makes no difference. There is no more, no less, magic in exercise at dawn than later in the day or at night. Each of us will find his own best time.

You don't have to join a gymnasium or a health club to start this program, nor must you rush out and buy expensive equipment. I almost wish you did—for then you would have made a financial commitment that you'd have to live up to.

Instead, you start in your own home, wherever you decide to. But you must decide to fit the program *into,* not on top of, your present schedule. If it is only tacked on to your day's activities, then it can be pulled off. By reviewing your recent use of time with the following questionnaire, you will be able to find where to slip these thirty minute sessions right into the middle of your day.

YOUR "TIME FOR FITNESS" QUESTIONNAIRE

Honestly and accurately recall where you were yesterday. Search for a half hour, three times a week, that you won't miss, where these exercises will refresh you most. It does not have to be the same half-hour each day. Let's see where it should go:

What time do you get up each morning on weekdays? On Saturday? On Sunday?

Did you feel refreshed when you got up?

Did you have breakfast immediately—or would you welcome a half-hour exercise period to really wake you up on Saturday or Sunday?

Can you get in one exercise period per week before breakfast?

*   *   *   *   *

How many coffee and rest breaks do you take each working day?

What do you do with these breaks?

How long a lunch period do you have?

How do you use this time?

Can you get in one exercise period per week during lunch time or in the afternoon—for instance, before going to the club for a game of golf?

*   *   *   *   *

What time do you leave work?

Do you need a drink to "unwind" when you get home?

How tired do you feel when you get home?

How did you spend the evening?

What time do you go to bed?

Can you get in one exercise period per week before bedtime to help you sleep better?

Why do most of us really feel tired in the evening? Because we have spent the whole day monotonously sitting. We rush home, to lie down—rest up—before bedtime. Too often our motto seems to be: don't stand if you can sit; don't sit if you can lie down.

Perhaps this is why the commonest phrase heard in funeral parlors is, "He looks so natural."

Every day that you increase your fitness you will gain mental tranquility and physical vigor. You will make more of all your natural gifts—mental and physical.

But you can only find this out by starting, so why not start today!

Appendix

A. CAUSES OF DEATH IN PROFESSIONAL MEN

Arteriosclerosis   All Others   Accidents   Cancer

Arteriosclerosis and other heart diseases   2085
Cancer   505
Accidents   91
All Others   584 + = 614
Done through personal computation of obituary notices
found in weekly publications of the J.A.M.A. for 1961.
Notice the overwhelming ratio of heart disease to all other
causes.

B. HEART ATTACKS DON'T WAIT FOR OLD AGE

Heart attacks show up as the major cause of death in our
highest earning years.

Age	Number of Deaths from Heart Attacks				
30's	14				
40's		93			
50's			220		
60's				267	
70's					274
80's			158		
90's	24				

Total number of deaths 1050

A proper fitness program can push this chart back as much
as forty years.

C. BLOOD PRESSURE AND LIFE EXPECTANCY

The accompanying chart will give you an opportunity to see the approximate life expectancy you currently can hope to have.

This chart is valid only if you are not significantly overweight. It begins with those who have a normal blood pressure of 120/80.

As you can see from this study, small elevations in blood pressure above this normal reading pose grave threats to our life expectancy.

Added weight also decreases our chance for longevity as shown in the chart on page 97.

Even worse, if overweight and blood pressure are combined, they increase our chances of a fatal stroke or heart attack to *more than double* those chances of persons who have only one of these disorders.

A proper fitness program, as described in this book, will combat both high blood pressure and overweight. Why not start that program—today!

D. POSSIBILITIES OF LIFE EXPECTANCY *

Blood Pressure	Remaining Years	Reduction of Life Expectancy Years Lost
At age 35		
Normal	41½	
130/90	37½	4
140/95	32½	9
150/100	25	16½
At age 45		
Normal	32	
130/90	29	3
140/95	26	6
150/100	20½	11½
At age 55		
Normal	23½	
130/90	22½	1
140/95	19½	4
150/100	17½	6

* Metropolitan Life Insurance Co. "Statistical Data from 28 Insurance companies" 1961.

E. THE AMAZING STORY OF MR. MARATHON

No individual ever demonstrated the benefits of vigorous running and exercise better than "Mr. Marathon." A renowned long distance runner from the Boston area, he suffered an untimely death at the age of 69. Five years before he died he was told that he had a cancer of the large intestine, but he refused to have anything done about it for three years. When he finally consented to surgery it was no longer possible to remove the entire malignancy and it eventually claimed his life.

Because of his past as a long distance runner many were interested in the condition of his heart and arteries. An autopsy showed that his coronary arteries, the arteries to his heart, were about five times larger than those of the average man.

This was not due to some inborn abnormality, but caused by his training and exercise program. Despite the fact that he had not avoided hardening of the arteries, but had about the same number of hard placques in his arteries as anyone else at this age would be expected to have, these were of far less a problem to his circulation than is usually the case. Since the channels of his circulation were so large these hard areas would only cause a ripple in the stream, while in the average person they could be reducing the blood flow to a half or a third of its normal volume.

Every one of us can create this type of increased capacity in our own circulation through vigorous exercise. By doing so, we dramatically reduce the chances of a heart attack or stroke.